INFLUENZA

**Recent Titles in the
Biographies of Disease Series**

Parkinson's Disease
Nutan Sharma

Depression
Blaise A. Aguirre

Diabetes
Andrew Galmer

Stroke
Jonathan A. Edlow

INFLUENZA

Roni K. Devlin

Biographies of Disease
Julie K. Silver, M.D., Series Editor

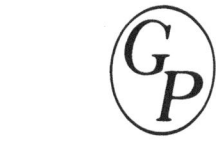

GREENWOOD PRESS
Westport, Connecticut • London

Library of Congress Cataloging-in-Publication Data

Devlin, Roni K., 1968–
   Influenza / Roni K. Devlin.
      p. ; cm.—(Biographies of disease, ISSN 1940-445X)
   Includes bibliographical references and index.
   ISBN 978-0-313-34259-2 (alk. paper)
   1. Influenza—History—Popular works. 2. Influenza—Popular works. I. Title. II.
Series.
   [DNLM: 1. Influenza, Human. WC 515 D497i 2008]
   RC150.1.D48   2008
   616.20′3—dc22   2008028510

British Library Cataloguing in Publication Data is available.

Copyright © 2008 by Roni K. Devlin

Library of Congress Catalog Card Number: 2008028510
ISBN: 978-0-313-34259-2
ISSN: 1940-445X

First published in 2008

Greenwood Press, 88 Post Road West, Westport, CT 06881
An imprint of Greenwood Publishing Group, Inc.
www.greenwood.com

Printed in the United States of America

The paper used in this book complies with the
Permanent Paper Standard issued by the National
Information Standards Organization (Z39.48–1984).

10 9 8 7 6 5 4 3 2 1

I dedicate this book to my mother, Jeri Lynn Devlin, who has,
without a doubt, been the biggest source of encouragement throughout
my medical and writing careers. May we continue on the path of literary
endeavors together for years to come.

Roni K. Devlin, M.D.
March 2008

Contents

Figures   ix

Series Foreword   xi

Preface   xiii

Introduction   xv

Chapter 1. The Influenza Virus   1
Definition of a Virus   1
Discovery of the Influenza Virus   4
Classification and Morphology of the Influenza Virus   12
Viral Pathogenicity and Host Responses   16

Chapter 2. The Epidemiology of Influenza   21
Definitions and Timelines   21
Influenza Antigenic Drift and Shift   25
Significance of Influenza Strain H5N1   27

Chapter 3. The Influenza Pandemic of 1918   31
Description of the Pandemic   32
Global Influence of the Pandemic   43

Factors Influencing Severity of Disease	49
Significance of the Pandemic for Today	54
Preparation for a Future Influenza Pandemic	55
Chapter 4. The Clinical Manifestations of Influenza	59
Uncomplicated Influenza	60
Complicated Influenza	62
Extra-Pulmonary Complications of Influenza	65
Influenza Manifestations in Special Patient Populations	68
Chapter 5. Making the Diagnosis of Influenza	71
Clinical Diagnosis of Influenza	71
Laboratory Diagnosis of Influenza	79
Future Development of Diagnostic Tests for Influenza	84
Chapter 6. Treatment and Prevention of Influenza	85
Treatments for Influenza	87
Prevention of Influenza	95
Areas of Future Research for Treatment and Prevention of Influenza	105
Conclusions	107
Timeline	111
Glossary	119
Bibliography	125
Index	129

Figures

Figure 1.1. Pfeiffer's Bacillus   6

Figure 1.2. Portrait of Richard Shope   9

Figure 1.3. Portrait of Christopher H. Andrewes   10

Figure 1.4. Electron Micrograph of Influenza A   14

Figure 1.5. Electron Micrograph of Influenza C   16

Figure 2.1. Electron Micrograph of Avian Influenza H5N1   27

Figure 3.1. U.S. Army Field Hospital, No. 29   35

Figure 3.2. U.S. Army Camp Hospital, No. 45   36

Figure 3.3. Preventative Treatment against Influenza   42

Figure 3.4. Self-Portrait with Bent Head, 1912   46

Figure 4.1. Pulmonary Autopsy Specimen, 1918   63

Figure 5.1. Inoculation of Embryonic Chicken Eggs   82

Figure 6.1. Emergency Hospital for Influenza Patients   86

Figure 6.2. Variola (Smallpox) Virus   96

Figure 6.3. Modified Smallpox   97

Figure 6.4. Influenza Vaccination Cartoon   99

Figure 6.5. Swine Flu Vaccination   103

Series Foreword

Every disease has a story to tell: about how it started long ago and began to disable or even take the lives of its innocent victims, about the way it hurts us, and about how we are trying to stop it. In this *Biographies of Disease* series, the authors tell the stories of the diseases that we have come to know and dread.

The stories of these diseases have all of the components that make for great literature. There is incredible drama played out in real-life scenes from the past, present, and future. You'll read about how men and women of science stumbled trying to save the lives of those they aimed to protect. Turn the pages and you'll also learn about the amazing success of those who fought for health and won, often saving thousands of lives in the process.

If you don't want to be a health professional or research scientist now, when you finish this book you may think differently. The men and women in this book are heroes who often risked their own lives to save or improve ours. This is the biography of a disease, but it is also the story of real people who made incredible sacrifices to stop it in its tracks.

Julie K. Silver, M.D.
Assistant Professor, Harvard Medical School
Department of Physical Medicine and Rehabilitation

Preface

In my work as an infectious disease physician, I am asked daily to provide care to patients with a variety of symptoms thought to be the result of infection with bacteria, viruses, fungi, or parasites. I am no stranger, therefore, to influenza, as both a viral entity and a distinguishable clinical disease state. It is an honor for me to be the chosen author of this book, and I hope that I can convey my interest in the organism, the disease it causes, and the historical importance of its presence to the reader of this series. The *Biographies of Disease* series is a perfect concept in which to explore influenza, because the virus has existed for centuries; continues to cause seasonal outbreaks with, as of yet, no cure; and will likely be the cause of a potentially devastating pandemic in the future. By approaching the virus and its disease process from a biographical perspective, we may better understand how the history of influenza and the significance of its past influence the hope for prevention and treatment of the illness in the future.

Much of the material found in this book has been obtained through my years of training as a physician, as well as through additional targeted review and research. *Influenza* contains much information, as well as aids designed to assist in understanding the material, including the following:

- a list of illustrations, including descriptive captions
- an introduction that explains the evolution of thought leading to the "germ theory," which eventually allowed advancement of the scientific study of infectious agents and the discovery of the influenza virus
- six narrative chapters on topics related to influenza, as follows:

  - Chapter 1 introduces the viral entity, the discovery of the influenza virus, and the characteristics of the influenza virus and its hosts that lead to its pathogenicity.
  - The epidemiology of influenza is explored in detail in Chapter 2, including a specific discussion of the avian influenza strain H5N1.
  - The influenza pandemic of 1918 is the specific subject of Chapter 3, and it is explored in detail with regard to its history, its global influence, and its significance for the influenza risks of today.
  - Additional details of the clinical manifestations of influenza are discussed in Chapter 4.
  - Methods of diagnosis used by today's healthcare providers are covered in Chapter 5.
  - Chapter 6 focuses on the prevention and treatment options currently available for influenza, with a brief mention of areas in need of future research.

- a conclusion chapter, reiterating the important points in the understanding of influenza, including the tendency of the virus to mutate and the concern for a future pandemic
- a collection of tables and sidebars with additional facts, comments, and statistics to complement the text
- a comprehensive timeline of significant events occurring in the history of influenza
- a glossary with concise definitions of important terms
- a bibliography, which should provide the reader with access to works that were of interest and help in the writing of this manuscript
- an alphabetized index, for easy search of subjects discussed in the work

Introduction

Each disease has a nature of its own, and none arises without its natural cause.

Hippocrates, Physician, 400 B.C.

Hippocrates (460–377 B.C.), a Greek physician now known as the "Father of Medicine," was one of the first healers to propose that diseases have both a natural cause and a natural cure. Although the concept may not seem particularly outrageous now, it was of monumental importance in Hippocrates' time, because illnesses were most often attributed to religious or supernatural causes. Hippocrates is thought to be responsible for a collection of writings called the *Hippocratic Corpus*, approximately seventy separate works covering many aspects of medicine, from both the professional and patient perspectives. Along with his novel theories of disease, Hippocrates' writings (and teachings, as he also founded a medical school) put particular emphasis on the doctor-patient relationship. One of the manuscripts contained in the *Hippocratic Corpus* is known as the "Hippocratic Oath," a pledge taken by physicians to practice medicine in a humane, ethical, and compassionate manner. A modernized version of the Hippocratic Oath is now recited by most students on graduation from medical school.

The Hippocratic Oath

I swear by Apollo Physician and Asclepius and Hygieia and Panaceia and all the gods and goddesses, making them my witnesses, that I will fulfill according to my ability and judgment this oath and this covenant:

To hold him who has taught me this art as equal to my parents and to live my life in partnership with him, and if he is in need of money to give him a share of mine, and to regard his offspring as equal to my brothers in male lineage and to teach them this art—if they desire to learn it—without fee and covenant; to give a share of precepts and oral instruction and all the other learning to my sons and to the sons of him who has instructed me and to pupils who have signed the covenant and have taken an oath according to the medical law, but no one else.

I will apply dietetic measures for the benefit of the sick according to my ability and judgment; I will keep them from harm and injustice.

I will neither give a deadly drug to anybody who asked for it, nor will I make a suggestion to this effect. Similarly I will not give to a woman an abortive remedy. In purity and holiness I will guard my life and my art.

I will not use the knife, not even on sufferers from stone, but will withdraw in favor of such men as are engaged in this work.

Whatever houses I may visit, I will come for the benefit of the sick, remaining free of all intentional injustice, of all mischief and in particular of sexual relations with both female and male persons, be they free or slaves.

What I may see or hear in the course of the treatment or even outside of the treatment in regard to the life of men, which on no account one must spread abroad, I will keep to myself, holding such things shameful to be spoken about.

If I fulfill this oath and do not violate it, may it be granted to me to enjoy life and art, being honored with fame among all men for all time to come; if I transgress it and swear falsely, may the opposite of all this be my lot.

In addition to his extensive teachings and writings, Hippocrates is also credited with many clinical discoveries. He is thought to be one of the first to describe an illness suggestive of influenza in 412 B.C. Other similar descriptions of an illness thought to be influenza were found written on paper dating back to the Middle Ages. In the fifteenth century, the term "influenza" was first used to describe the clinical syndrome, and it referred to a disease attributed to the "influence of the heavens." The word was adopted into English in the eighteenth century, about the same time as the French named the disease "la grippe." Today, people often just refer to it as "the flu." The disease, by whatever name, and the pathogen that causes it are the topics of the following pages.

Interestingly, although the disease process of influenza has been clearly described throughout history since the days of Hippocrates, there was a long

Important Names in the Evolution of Germ Theory

Hippocrates (460–377 B.C.): A Greek physician, now known as the Father of Medicine, who described a clinical illness thought to be influenza in 412 B.C. He believed in the natural cause and cure of diseases and was a great educator in the field of medicine. He is thought to be the original author of the *Hippocratic Oath*.

Empedocles (495–435 B.C.): A Greek physician, philosopher, and poet who initially proposed the elemental theory.

Aristotle (384–322 B.C.): A Greek philosopher who contributed to refinement of the elemental theory and linked classical elements with certain individual temperaments.

Galen (131–201 B.C.): A Greek physician who treated both gladiators and emperors during his medical career. He was a proponent of dissection as a means of understanding anatomy and disease processes. He also aided in refinement of the ill humour theory.

William Farr (1807–1883): A statistician named as assistant commissioner for the 1851 London census. He believed in the miasma theory.

Florence Nightingale (1820–1910): A nurse and a believer in the benefits of sanitation practices to combat the effects of miasma.

Sir Edward Chadwick (1800–1890): A proponent of the miasma theory, he became a sanitation reformer in England.

Sir John Simon (1816–1904): The first Medical Officer of Health for London, who attributed the cause of disease to miasma.

Justus von Liebig (1803–1873): A German chemist who was a proponent of the blood generation theory.

Louis Pasteur (1822–1895): A French chemist who was responsible for many discoveries in both science and medicine; he was instrumental in establishing the germ theory of disease.

Robert Koch (1843–1910): A German physician and researcher who proposed a set of criteria that firmly established the validity of the germ theory of disease.

Charles Chamberland (1851–1908): A colleague of Pasteur and inventor of a filter used to confirm the presence of infectious agents smaller than bacteria.

period in which humankind did not realize that microscopic germs were the causative agents of infectious diseases. Indeed, theories involving elements, ill humours, divine judgment, miasma, and spontaneous blood generation were generally accepted, and the practices for diagnosis, treatment, and prevention of disease reflected these beliefs. To fully understand the biography of influenza, it is necessary to review the evolution of thought that eventually led to acceptance of the "germ theory."

The "elemental theory," proposed initially by Empedocles (495–435 B.C.), a physician, philosopher, and poet, suggested that four "elements" were responsible for the fundamental constituents of all nature, and that those elements were manifestations of essential physical qualities. For example, water represented wetness and coldness, earth personified dryness and coldness, air was related to wetness and hotness, and fire embodied dryness and hotness. Aristotle (384–322 B.C.), the well-known Greek philosopher, and subsequent other authors who were proponents of Hippocratic teachings, refined the elemental theory and associated it with certain "temperaments" of individuals. Eventually, it evolved into the more detailed "ill humour theory."

A Greek physician named Galen (131–201 B.C.), known for his treatment of gladiators in Pergamos and, later, the care of Emperor Marcus Aurelius and his son Commodus in Rome, is now credited with many intriguing ideas in the practice of medicine. He was a proponent of dissection as a means to fully understand anatomy (indeed, some of his original statements concerning human anatomy, inferred from his dissection of animals, were later proven false when human cadavers were finally able to be studied in detail), and he was known to have performed fairly bold surgical interventions in his time. Galen is also credited with refining the ill humour theory. The theory proposed that the four classic elements entered the body through food, drink, and atmosphere, and that these were converted in specific organs to four fluids, or humours. A balance of such humours was necessary for good health. Linked to their corresponding elements, the four humours were as follows:

- earth: black bile
- water: phlegm
- air: blood
- fire: yellow bile

As before, physical qualities were associated with each element and its corresponding humour. For example, the cold and wet months of winter were thought to contribute to production of phlegm, leading to cough and lung problems. The heat and dryness of summer, in contrast, shifted the humoural balance to yellow bile, leading to digestive diseases such as diarrhea and dysentery.

Each humour was also thought to be associated with a particular temperament, as follows:

- black bile: melancholic
- phlegm: phlegmatic
- blood: sanguine
- yellow bile: choleric

The Four Humours and Their Corresponding Temperaments		
Black bile	Melancholic	Thoughtful, kind, considerate of others, highly creative, obsessive, prone to depression, perfectionist, introspective, sentimental
Phlegm	Phlegmatic	Calm, self-content, shy, resistant to change, consistent, relaxed, rational, curious, observant, reliable, compassionate, sluggish, cowardly, lazy
Blood	Sanguine	Arrogant, cocky, indulgent, confident, impulsive, unpredictable, outgoing, amorous, happy, generous, optimistic
Yellow bile	Choleric	Ambitious, energetic, passionate, dominant, quick to anger, bad-tempered, violent, vengeful

Practices such as dietary manipulations, ingestions of potions and emetics, and bloodletting (sometimes using leeches) were used to keep the humours in balance, and it was thought that following proper behavior with regard to personal habits and diet would allow an individual to avoid most diseases. The astrological signs of the zodiac were also thought to be associated with certain humours, and, even today, certain personality traits are thought to correlate with specific astrological signs, which are determined by the configuration of the stars and planets at the time of an individual's birth.

Despite Hippocrates' teachings that a natural disease process may have a corresponding natural cure, the previously described Greco-Roman theories of disease were also influenced by the beliefs in multiple gods. New theories based on the concept of divine judgment were more widely accepted as Christianity became a recognized religion. In essence, outbreaks and epidemics (such as medieval plague or sweating sickness) were presumed to be the result of God's wrath on people or populations who strayed from the presumed path of righteousness. Another religious emphasis was the association of disease and the "unclean." From the Middle Ages into the mid-1800s, the "miasma theory" dominated the European discussion of disease process. With little in the way of available sanitation practices and the continued movement of people from rural areas into crowded cities, the stench and debris (including fecal matter) of the time were overwhelming. The miasma theory postulated that the air could become infested with a contagious "influence" when combined with decomposing organic matter from the earth. The resulting vapor, or miasma, was thought to be responsible for disease. For much of the 1800s, outbreaks of diseases such as plague and cholera were attributed to miasma. Many significant scientists, physicians, and researchers in history were proponents of the miasma theory. William Farr (1807–1883), the famous statistician and assistant commissioner for the 1851 London census, thought miasma from the River Thames caused cholera. Florence Nightingale (1820–1910), known for her nursing work during the Crimean War, strove to make hospitals sanitary and "fresh-smelling" as a result of her miasma beliefs. Sir Edwin Chadwick (1800–1890), a great sanitation reformer, and Sir John Simon (1816–1904), the first Medical Officer of Health for London, were also proponents of the miasma theory.

Another theory that existed in the 1800s was based on the belief that there could be spontaneous generation of disease within the blood. The "blood generation theory" did not propose that a contagion caused disease within the blood, but rather that a spontaneous "fermentation" or chemical process occurring in the blood was responsible for illness. German chemist Justus von Liebig (1803–1873) was a major supporter of this theory, but much of the scientific community chose to side with the miasma believers at the time.

Despite the fact that it had been proposed previously in scientific writings that diseases could be the result of transfer of microscopic agents from outside the body, it was not until the late 1800s that the "germ theory" was formulated. Louis Pasteur (1822–1895), a French chemist, was instrumental in providing evidence that germs existed. During his experimentations, he determined (by using a microscope) that germs were responsible for souring beverages such as wine, beer, and milk (a phenomenon now known as fermentation). He also showed that such germs could be removed from the liquids by first boiling and then cooling the solution. This technique is now called pasteurization.

The germ theory was further refined with the work of Robert Koch (1843–1910). A German physician, Koch traveled to an area known as Wollenstein to become District Medical Officer in 1872. While there, Koch realized that many regional farm animals were dying of a disease called anthrax. Earlier scientists had identified an anthrax bacterium but had yet to provide proof that it was responsible for the actual disease. Creating a rudimentary laboratory in his home and using a microscope given to him by his wife, Koch began to study anthrax. He obtained tissue from animals that were sick with the disease and, via homemade wooden splinters, inoculated the specimens into healthy mice; these mice ultimately died of anthrax. He then took material from healthy animals and inoculated samples into new mice; these mice remained healthy. Finally, Koch was able to grow pure cultures of the anthrax bacteria by using the aqueous material of an ox's eye.

Koch eventually published his results, and continued his microbiology work in a number of different settings. He later was able to identify and isolate the bacterium responsible for tuberculosis, and the organism that causes cholera.

In 1884, Koch formulated a set of criteria designed to establish a link between an infectious agent and a disease process; it was further refined in 1890. Koch's postulates are as follows:

1. The infectious agent must be found in every case of the disease and in such a relationship to the damaged tissue as to explain the damage.
2. The infectious agent must be isolated from a diseased organism and grown in pure culture outside the body of its host.
3. The cultured agent, when introduced into a healthy animal, must produce a disease that is identical in its characteristics to the naturally occurring disease.
4. The microorganism must be able to be isolated from the inoculated, diseased experimental host and proven identical to the original infecting agent.

Although not all organisms adhere strictly to Koch's postulates, the criteria continue to guide scientists and researchers in their work as they attempt to identify the causative agents in today's emerging infectious diseases. Not surprisingly, Koch was awarded the Nobel Prize for Medicine in 1905.

Once the germ theory became widely accepted, and Koch's postulates were available to guide work being done with regard to infectious diseases, additional research attempting to isolate agents of infection was pursued with vigor. Despite the impressive work linking different bacteria to certain diseases, however, there remained many illnesses that were thought likely to be caused by germs for which no infecting bacterium could be found. In fact, even the concept of vaccination, now a primary technique used in the prevention of many illnesses, was proven by experimentation over one hundred years before viruses were even identified as agents of disease. In the late nineteenth century, Charles Chamberland (1851–1908), a colleague of Pasteur, developed an unglazed porcelain filter that trapped bacteria but allowed smaller, infectious particles to pass through. Botanists, using Chamberland's filter, found that diseases could be transmitted to healthy plants by inoculating them with the liquid that remained after filtration of samples from infected plants; the small particles in the filtrate were initially called *contagium vivum fluidum*, meaning "soluble living germ." Ultimately, such infectious agents were given the name virus (Latin for "slimy liquid" or "poison"). With additional experimentation, scientists were eventually able to show that filterable agents, or viruses, were also the cause of human diseases, including polio and yellow fever. It was only a matter of time, of course, until a virus was discovered as the cause of influenza.

Important Facts about Influenza

According to the Centers for Disease Control (CDC) in Atlanta, Georgia, influenza affects up to 60 million children and adults in the United States each year. Surveillance of influenza activity revealed an annual average of approximately 36,000 deaths during 1990–1999 and 226,000 hospitalizations during 1979–2001 in the United States alone.

Per the CDC, approximately 10–20% of the world's population is affected by seasonal influenza, with an estimated 3–5 million cases of severe disease each year; worldwide, 250,000–500,000 deaths are attributed to influenza annually.

In addition to the morbidity and mortality it causes, influenza also has a substantial economic impact. A report published by the World Health Organization (WHO) in 2003 revealed that influenza outbreaks imposed a burden of US $5,000 million per year on the U.S. economy because of hospital and other healthcare costs and lost productivity, as estimated in 1986.

Amazingly, influenza, the virus and the clinical syndrome that has existed for centuries and has been the subject of much medical and scientific research, still causes significant grief for humankind.

It is considered fairly certain within the medical community that a significant, worldwide pandemic of influenza will occur sometime in the future, despite the current understanding of the virus and the ongoing attempts to control it. It has been postulated that the global mortality of such a pandemic could be as high as 62 million deaths. It is thus the goal of this book to enlighten the reader about influenza, as both a viral pathogen and a disease entity capable of causing great damage and death. By understanding the influenza virus and the characteristics that influence its ability to cause disease, one can further comprehend the factors involved in large outbreaks that have previously been called "the greatest medical holocaust in history" (Waring, 1971, p. 33). Influenza is a fascinating virus, and the disease it causes will continue to be the focus of much discussion, research, and scholarly activity. Perhaps with this biographical exploration of influenza, a full understanding of the virus' role throughout the world's history will help with answers to questions about the implications of the disease for the future.

1

The Influenza Virus

vi-rus—one of a group of minute infectious agents, with certain excep-
tions (e.g., poxviruses) not resolved in the light microscope, and characterized by a lack of independent metabolism and by the ability to
replicate only within living host cells. Like living organisms, they are able
to reproduce with genetic continuity and the possibility of mutation.

Defintion, *Dorland's Illustrated Medical Dictionary*, 2007

DEFINITION OF A VIRUS

Viruses are actually quite distinct from other infectious agents such
as bacteria, fungi, or parasites. Bacteria are the oldest forms of life
on earth and are one-celled living organisms that typically multiply by cell division. Despite being unicellular, bacteria come in many
shapes and sizes. They are ubiquitous and exist in virtually every environ-
ment, including on and in the human body. Although bacteria are instrumental in maintaining the balance of the global ecosystem, they have also
been the cause of some of the most deadly diseases in the history of
humankind, such as the bubonic plague, cholera, leprosy, and syphilis.
Humans can live in harmony with many bacteria, but some strains, such as

Streptococcus pneumoniae and *Staphylococcus aureus*, still cause terrible disease, devastation, and even death.

Fungi can exist as molds or yeast and are in the same microbiological domain, *Eukaryota*, as plants and animals. Fungi, which are quite diverse, generally lack chlorophyll, have a cell wall, and can reproduce either sexually or asexually. Humans often have a symbiotic, or shared, relationship with fungi, although some fungi are unfortunately pathogenic and cause human illness, such as ringworm.

Parasites, conversely, are simple organisms (either plant or animal) that exist either in or on another living entity, often at some cost to the host. Parasites can cause a variety of diseases, including hookworm and scabies in humans.

Perhaps the most striking difference between bacteria, fungi, or parasites and viruses is, of course, that viruses are not considered by most scientists to be alive. They do not eat, drink, have sex, or produce waste. They are simply genetic material surrounded by an enveloping substance that allows the virus to enter a host. Usually, the surrounding substance has to be removed for the virus to cause disease. Examples of human diseases caused by viruses include acquired immunodeficiency syndrome (AIDS), chicken pox, hepatitis, and polio. Viruses are also able to infect other biological organisms, including animals and even bacteria themselves. The viruses that infect bacteria are called bacteriophages (or simply phages), and they are currently a topic of much study and discussion because it is hoped that phages might be able to be used as treatments to target specific bacterial strains that act as human pathogens.

The exact origin of viruses on earth is not known. There are several theories that might explain their existence, however. One hypothesis suggests that viruses may be the result of "escaped" pieces of genetic material that originally came from a living organism. A second hypothesis is that viruses were derived from living cells that "devolved" through a streamlining process known as reverse evolution. Another view suggests that viruses originated as a primitive molecule capable of replication, implying that more advanced life forms could have evolved from them. Specifically, the influenza virus was found first in birds, although the disease caused in the avian host is quite different than that found in humans. Unfortunately, humans can become infected with an avian virus if enough of an exposure occurs, but it is unusual for an avian influenza to spread from person to person. This concept becomes important with regard to the future threat of avian influenza as cause of a human pandemic and will be discussed further in later chapters.

Regardless of its origin, a viral particle, or virion, essentially exists for one purpose: to make more viruses. Despite this singular goal, viruses are not able to reproduce on their own. They must invade a host and use the host cell's mechanisms to make new viral particles. A virus, then, is simply a carrier for genes, nicely surrounded by a protective layer. The surrounding coat can come in a variety of shapes, and this allows for identification of four main categories of virus based on morphology: helical, icosahedral, enveloped, and complex. Influenza is an enveloped virus. Interestingly, in addition to allowing the viral particle to reach the desired target cell type, the type of surrounding coat actually plays a role in determining how a virus is transmitted between hosts. Envelopes that are made up of fats are easily broken down outside the body. Viruses with this type of shell must be transmitted with the aid of respiratory secretions, blood, or body (i.e., sexual) fluids. Influenza, then, is spread from person to person in aerosolized droplets that are expelled from the respiratory tract during coughing, sneezing, or even talking. Transmission requires fairly close contact, because the droplets do not remain suspended in the air for long, and they generally travel only a short distance through the air. The influenza virus can remain infectious if settled on a hard surface for up to two days; this allows transfer of the droplet-encased virus by hand-to-mouth or hand-to-nose contact. Viruses without such packaging are more stable outside their host and are usually transmitted by the "fecal-oral" route. This implies that the host comes in contact with fecal matter (on unwashed hands or food, for instance) and then transmits the virus, hiding within this fecal material, to the mouth. From here, the virus is ingested and then travels to its desired location in the body to start the disease process. Examples of disease processes that are caused by fecal-oral viral transmission are polio and certain types of hepatitis.

The genetic material found in viruses can come in a variety of shapes and sizes and is made of either ribonucleic acid (RNA) or deoxyribonucleic acid (DNA). RNA is a strand of genes comprised of chemicals within a backbone, held together with ribose sugars and phosphates. There are four different chemicals that can be found in RNA: adenine, guanine, cytosine, and uracil. RNA can be structured as a single-stranded or a double-stranded molecule and can exist in several forms, including messenger RNA (mRNA), transfer RNA, ribosomal RNA, noncoding RNA, and catalytic RNA. Each of these different RNA types has a specific function, but all serve to aid in the synthesis of proteins.

DNA, conversely, uses deoxyribose sugars and phosphates to complement its backbone, which may form a single or a double strand. The four chemicals found in DNA are cytosine, guanine, adenine, and thymine (compared with uracil found in RNA). The DNA backbone also carries genetic information like RNA, but the DNA sequence must be copied into a complementary RNA sequence before protein synthesis can occur; this process is called transcription. Translation, or production of proteins from the genetic code in the RNA copy, can then follow. Also, if the genetic instructions dictate, a host cell may simply

> ### Role of RNA in Viral Replication
>
> A host cell contains ribosomes, made of proteins and ribosomal RNA. Ribosomes are the sites in which protein synthesis actually occurs, and it is messenger RNA that carries information from DNA to the ribosome. Once messenger RNA is bound to a ribosome, it is translated into a protein form; this process requires the help of transfer RNA, which moves a specific amino acid to a growing protein chain. Noncoding RNA is not translated directly into proteins but may play a role in regulating other genes involved in the translation process. Catalytic RNA may participate in chemical reactions, including cutting of the bond between amino acid sequences found within the ribosome. All of these activities occur as the result of a viral infection: once a virus has successfully entered a host cell, it simply uses its genetic code to control the cell's process of protein synthesis, allowing its own replication to occur at the expense of the cell's usual activities.

copy its genome in a process called DNA replication and forego protein synthesis altogether.

It is the sequence of the four chemicals within the strands of RNA and DNA that acts as a blueprint, or template, for the translation of the genetic code into proteins. The smallest viruses contain genes that will encode only a few different proteins, whereas large viruses might have the ability to encode several hundred. With its genetic material and the resulting proteins, a virus uses the host cell's own replication pathways to "reproduce," infect other cells, and thereby cause its ill effects. Whether RNA or DNA, the genetic code within a virion contains the map needed to outline the path to the particle's own replication. The purpose of this is, of course, to allow production and survival of its kind, a reasonable goal for any infectious agent. With regard to survival, influenza may be considered a very successful virus.

DISCOVERY OF THE INFLUENZA VIRUS

As a disease entity, influenza has been described and documented in the medical literature by physicians, researchers, and scientists for centuries. However, it was not until the mid-1900s that the influenza virus itself was discovered.

For many years, it was mistakenly thought that influenza was caused by a bacterium. In 1892, a German physician and bacteriologist named Richard Friedrich Johannes Pfeiffer (1858–1945) collected samples of mucus from sick patients who were thought to be suffering from influenza. From these specimens, he was able to identify a common, small, rod-shaped bacterium. He called this organism *Bacillus influenzae*, but it became more commonly known as Pfeiffer's

---

Important Names in Influenza History

Richard Friedrich Johannes Pfeiffer (1858–1945): A German physician and bacteriologist who identified a bacterium (called Pfeiffer's bacillus), mistakenly thought to be the cause of influenza.

Peter K. Olitsky (1886–1964) and Frederick L. Gates (1853–1929): Scientists at the Rockefeller Institute who used Chamberland's filter to look for the causative agent of influenza.

Charles Jules Henry Nicolle (1866–1936): French scientist at the Pasteur Institute who studied influenza in monkeys.

Richard Shope (1901–1966): American physician-scientist who identified the virus causing swine influenza and aided in the search for the viral cause of human influenza.

Paul Lewis (1879–1929): American physician-scientist who served as a mentor for Richard Shope.

Christopher H. Andrewes (1896–1988), Wilson Smith (1897–1965), and Patrick Laidlaw (1881–1940): English researchers who identified the influenza virus using ferret and, later, mice subjects.

---

bacillus (see Figure 1.1). Pfeiffer published a report claiming that his bacillus was the causative agent of influenza. This idea did not seem particularly unreasonable, in part because bacteria had been shown previously to cause other infectious diseases such as cholera and bubonic plague. Of note, just before his work with influenza, Pfeiffer acted as the assistant to Robert Koch at the Institute of Hygiene in Berlin from 1887 to 1891. Koch was the physician who validated the germ theory and published the four postulates that continue to help guide research in infectious diseases. In the late 1890s, Pfeiffer worked again with Koch to investigate the plague in India and malaria in Italy.

Pfeiffer's theory that his bacillus was the cause of influenza was not seriously challenged until many years later. During subsequent disease outbreaks, in various parts of the world, researchers obtained samples of respiratory secretions from patients sick with influenza but could not always find evidence of Pfeiffer's bacillus. In 1918, as a pandemic with influenza began to be recognized, the illness reached Camp Lewis, Washington, as a troop ship arrived from Philadelphia. Scientists at Camp Lewis took mucus samples from their sick soldiers. Although the illness of many soldiers clearly fit with influenza, only a few specimens showed growth of Pfeiffer's bacillus, whereas some samples showed growth of other bacteria. It was concluded that the epidemic at Camp Lewis was not caused by *Bacillus influenzae*, and it was further suggested that influenza might not be caused by a single bacterium at all. By performing autopsies, other

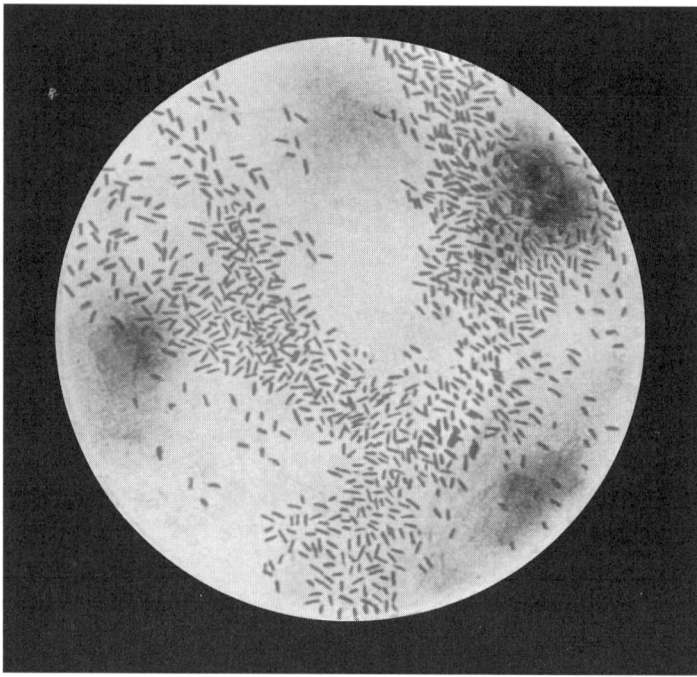

Figure 1.1. Pfeiffer's Bacillus. Photomicrograph of Pfeiffer's bacillus, now known as *Haemophilus influenzae*, as seen using Gram staining technique. Image used with permission, courtesy of the CDC.

medical researchers realized that the findings in the lungs of influenza patients were distinct from those findings described in the lungs of patients known to have died from bacterial respiratory diseases. The suspicion for a possible viral agent as the cause of influenza could not be ignored, despite considerable disagreement among highly respected medical personnel for years to come.

In the 1920s, two scientists named Peter K. Olitsky (1886–1964) and Frederick L. Gates (1853–1929), working at the Rockefeller Institute for Medical Research, revisited a technique described previously by Chamberland. They took nasal secretions from patients thought to have the flu and passed the specimens through a porcelain filter. As before, the filters were designed to stop bacteria but would allow other smaller particles to pass through. The infectious agent in the secretions from influenza patients easily passed through the filters, suggesting that it was not a typical bacterium as Pfeiffer and others had previously thought. The organism identified initially by Olitsky and Gates was called *Bacterium pneumosintes*, and, although it was not a virus, it was small enough to pass through the filter. Olitsky and Gates attempted to study the organism using

---

Fascinating Facts about Pfeiffer

1880: Received his doctorate of medicine degree after attending the Kaiser-Wilhelms-Akademie in Berlin.

1887–1891: Acted as assistant to Robert Koch at the Institute of Hygiene in Berlin.

1892: Identified Pfeiffer's bacillus, a bacterium at one time thought to be the cause of influenza, now known as *Haemophilus influenzae*.

1894: Developed the technique of *bacteriolysis* (also known as Pfeiffer's phenomenon) using the cholera bacterium and guinea pig test subjects.

1896: Identified *Mycoplasma catarrhalis*, a bacterium known to cause respiratory diseases in humans.

1897: Traveled to India to study the plague under the guidance of Robert Koch.

1898: Traveled to Italy to study malaria under the guidance of Robert Koch.

1925: Retired as Emeritus Chair of Hygiene, Department of Science, at the Institute of Infectious Diseases in Breslan.

Koch's postulates. First, they injected pure cultures of the organism into the windpipes of rabbits and guinea pigs. The animals became ill with fever and, on autopsy, were found to have lesions in the lungs resembling that found in human influenza victims. Although their results were encouraging, their experiments were never able to be confirmed or duplicated by other scientists. It was finally discovered that the lung lesions in their animals had occurred as a result of the method of execution used in preparing the animals for autopsy, not because of the infecting organism. The search for the true causative agent of influenza continued.

Near the same time period, in Paris, Charles Jules Henry Nicolle (1866–1936) and colleagues at the Pasteur Institute filtered the respiratory secretions from an influenza patient and then injected the filtered material into the eyes and nose of two monkeys. The monkeys quickly developed a fever. They then administered the filtrate to a human volunteer via an injection under the skin. The volunteer also quickly became ill with symptoms consistent with influenza. Meanwhile, in Japan, researchers performed experiments on humans as the world was dealing with the great influenza pandemic of 1918. They inoculated the noses and throats of twelve healthy people with filtrated sputum from flu victims, the nose and throats of six healthy people with filtrated blood from flu victims, the subcutaneous tissue of four healthy people with filtrated flu sputum, and the subcutaneous tissue of four healthy persons with filtrated flu blood. As controls, they inoculated the noses and throats of fourteen healthy people with both pure and mixed bacterial preparations, including Pfeiffer's bacillus and streptococci. All of the subjects inoculated with infiltrates came down with influenza except those who had already experienced the flu during the pandemic. None of the subjects inoculated with the bacterial preparations became sick. With these studies in place, a virus as the cause of influenza seemed plausible.

A decade after Olitsky and Gates' filter experiment, a young doctor named Richard Shope (1901–1966) began to study influenza under the guidance of his mentor Paul Lewis (1879–1929) at the Rockefeller Institute. Lewis was a physician, born in Wisconsin but trained at the University of Pennsylvania, who was known for his passion and accomplishments in the laboratory; his previous work had been instrumental in the development of a polio vaccine. In 1929, a highly contagious respiratory illness was found to be spreading quickly through the swine on Iowa pig farms; a similar occurrence had been documented in 1918, as well, and smaller outbreaks occurred in autumn each year. Millions of pigs became ill with fever, runny noses, watery eyes, and respiratory symptoms. Thousands of pigs died during the outbreaks. Because of the clinical similarities to the human illness, the disease was called swine influenza.

Shope was born and bred on an Iowa farm and was the son of a doctor (see Figure 1.2). While attending Iowa State for college, he entered into premedical studies. He went on to finish his medical training in 1924 and joined the Rockefeller Institute as a researcher with an initial interest in tuberculosis, but his assignment in Iowa changed his course of study forever.

It occurred to Shope and Lewis that, perhaps in light of the similarities with regard to the outbreak timeline and the symptoms observed, the agent that caused the influenza pandemic of 1918 was now living in the pig population. Using Koch's postulates as a basis for experimentation, Shope quickly identified a bacterium in the secretions taken from infected pigs, and, interestingly, it resembled Pfeiffer's bacillus. Shope and Lewis named the organism *Hemophilus influenzae suis*. Next, this bacterium was inoculated into the noses of healthy pigs. Although the very first inoculated pig became ill, none of the pigs subsequently tested became sick. Shope and Lewis concluded that the bacterium could not be the agent responsible for swine influenza.

Sadly, in the midst of their investigations of swine influenza, Lewis became infected with the yellow fever virus while working in the laboratory during an outbreak in Brazil. After five days of progressive symptoms, he died from the infection. Shope, although clearly troubled by the death of his mentor, was determined to both finish the investigation he and Lewis had started and solve the mystery of swine influenza. Remembering the filter technique performed by Olitsky and Gates, he decided to look for a virus in the secretions of the

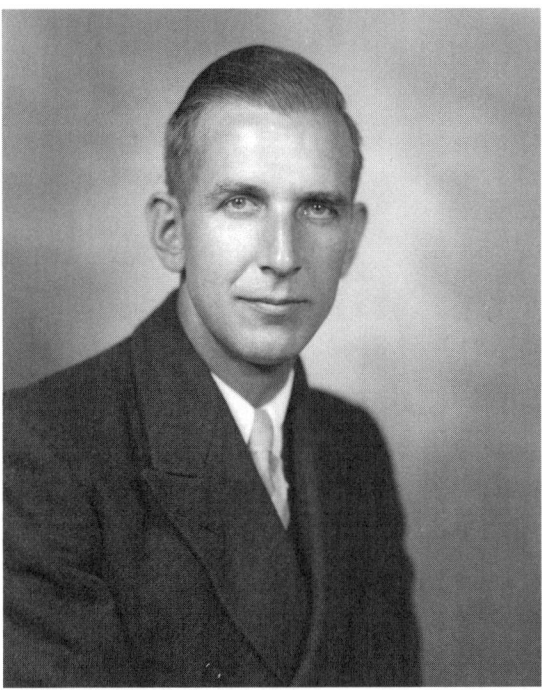

Figure 1.2. Portrait of Richard Shope. Courtesy of the Rockefeller Archive Center.

pigs sick with swine flu. Mucus was collected from sick pigs and then filtered. The collected filtrate was inoculated into the noses of healthy pigs. These pigs became sick with a mild, flu-like illness after injection. Then, Shope took both the filtrate and the *Hemophilus influenzae suis* bacterium and mixed them together. When this mixture was injected into healthy pigs, the swine became more severely ill with a full-blown influenza syndrome, including pneumonia. Shope concluded that the infectious agent causing swine influenza was in the filtered specimen (therefore likely a virus and not a bacterium), and that there might be a secondary infection in some pigs caused by the bacterium.

Around the same time, across the globe in the United Kingdom, a scientist named Christopher H. Andrewes (1896–1988) was recruited by the National Institute for Medical Research to help study influenza as part of the Medical Research Council (see Figure 1.3). Although medically trained as a physician, Andrewes was interested in laboratory research. He entered into the study of influenza with great enthusiasm, and his work was part of a lifelong career spent in conducting research with viruses.

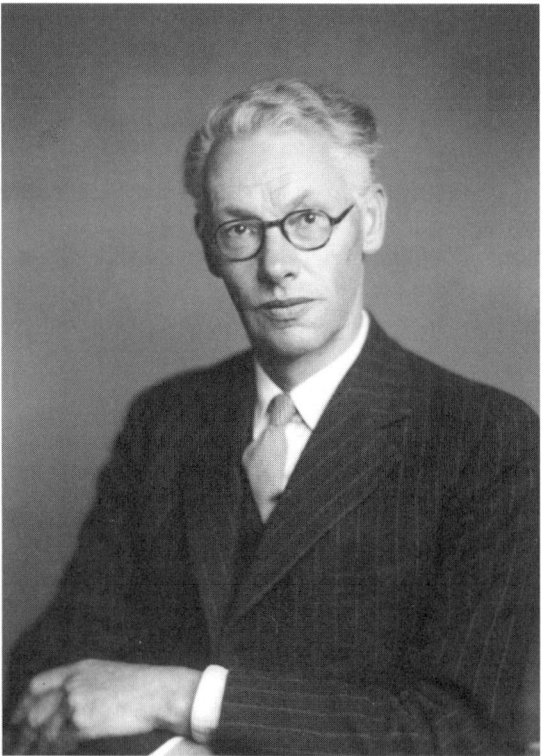

Figure 1.3. Portrait of Christopher H. Andrewes. Portrait credited to Walter Stone-man; used with permission from The Godfrey Argent Studio and The Royal Society, London, England.

Andrewes first became aware of viruses when he was a medical student in London at St. Bartholomew's Hospital. His father was professor of pathology there, and, on the top floor of the pathology wing, there was a scientist named Mervyn Gordon (1872–1953). Studying the vaccinia virus, as well as the mumps virus, while using a grant from the Medical Research Council, Gordon influenced Andrewes greatly with his enthusiasm for viral research. Andrewes went on to gain additional experience by traveling to New York in 1923 to study under Homer Swift (1881–1953) at the hospital of the Rockefeller Institute, followed by a return in 1925 to London to work with well-known researchers investigating the possible viral cause of fowl cancers. After this, Andrewes spent five years dividing his time between clinical medicine and laboratory research but ultimately joined the staff of the National Institute for Medical Research in 1927.

In 1933, an epidemic of influenza was identified in London and the surrounding area. Using Shope's techniques, Andrewes and his colleagues Wilson Smith (1897–1965) and Patrick Laidlaw (1881–1940) took filtered washings from sick patients and used them to inoculate two ferrets. (Ferrets were thought to be reasonable animals in the investigation of influenza because they had been successfully used in the study of distemper: they were susceptible to the disease, usually died when exposed to the disease, and seemed to exist well in cages. Unfortunately, they were also quick to bite and notably sharp-toothed, particularly when ill.) Once inoculated with the filtered washings from flu patients, the ferrets developed high fever, runny noses, and sneezing. Realizing that their investigations needed to be conducted with rigid laboratory techniques to ensure that their ferret subjects were not contracting the flu naturally, Andrewes and his colleagues developed a special facility in England where their ferrets lived in complete isolation; studies conducted at the facility confirmed their initial results. When Wilson Smith became ill with influenza after a sick ferret sneezed in his face, Andrewes isolated the viral strain and called it "WS." This strain was then used to inoculate future ferrets and is still available in the laboratory setting today.

Andrewes, Smith, and Laidlaw were quite successful in their studies with ferrets. They were able to conclude that a virus was present in filtered secretions, which could then be transmitted from human to ferret, from ferret to human (like in the case of the WS strain), and then from ferret to ferret. Interestingly, Pfeiffer's bacillus seemed to have little effect on the ferrets; the animals had the same disease whether inoculated with virus alone or with filtrate mixed with Pfeiffer's bacterium. Intrigued by each other's work, Shope and Andrewes met at Princeton and shared their data. Later, Andrewes noted that this was the beginning of a long and close friendship between the two men.

Ultimately, laboratory work revealed that mice could be infected with the influenza virus, and that these rodents were easier to study than the ferocious ferrets. Continuing his influenza work, Shope ultimately found that human and swine influenza viruses were not the same viral strain as he had originally thought. He found that the blood of pigs previously sick with swine influenza was only partially effective in preventing animals from becoming sick with human flu virus. This proved that the virus causing swine influenza and the virus causing human influenza were related but not identical, as he and Lewis had hypothesized earlier.

With the success of experiments performed on pigs, ferrets, and mice, Shope and Andrewes were ready to try their tests further on humans. They recruited volunteers of all ages in both the United States and England and collected blood samples from all subjects. Interestingly, the people who survived the flu in 1918 had antibodies that blocked infection from Shope's swine flu virus, whereas volunteers who had been born after 1918 did not have such antibodies. Other researchers collected field data, as well; patients sick in various outbreaks of influenza were routinely tested, and all were found to have the same virus. Interestingly, some patients tested during disease outbreaks suspected to be caused by influenza were found to be negative for the influenza virus; they were later found to have an illness caused by adenovirus, now known as one of the infecting agents of the common cold.

In the mid-1930s, two distinct viral strains were identified, named influenza A and influenza B. Influenza C was not identified until almost 1950. It is now known that influenza C tends to cause mild disease and is not likely of epidemiological significance to humans, whereas influenza B has been responsible for regional outbreaks in humankind (often every two to four years). Influenza A, however, has been the strain implicated in the major pandemics in history and is still the type most concerning for humans. Aquatic wild birds are the natural reservoir for avian influenza A, and they become infected with the virus through the gastrointestinal tract. Birds can leave behind viral particles in their droppings, which then easily contaminate water; once there, influenza viral particles may remain infectious for 100–200 days, depending on water temperature. Usually, avian influenza is not harmful to its bird host, but wide spread of the virus can easily occur because birds may travel for hundreds (or even thousands) of miles during migration. Recent identification of highly pathogenic strains of avian influenza in poultry has caused great concern for future potential of a devastating pandemic among humans, particularly with documentation of rapid viral evolution, an increasing tendency for the virus to be found in new host species (such as migratory birds and mammals), and confirmed geographic spread of the virus from Asia to Africa, Europe, and the Middle East.

Pigs may also play an important role in the biography of influenza. The respiratory tract of pigs contains receptors that bind both avian and human influenza viruses. It has been proposed that the genetic "reassortment" of avian and human influenza may occur in pigs, leading to a new and novel viral strain that can then be spread to mankind.

CLASSIFICATION AND MORPHOLOGY OF THE INFLUENZA VIRUS

Influenza has caused recurrent disease outbreaks for centuries, as has been well documented in our historical literature. Obviously, then, the virus has morphological characteristics that allow it to exist year after year. Medical technology has now advanced enough for researchers to further classify the influenza virus in terms of size, shape, and function.

Influenza belongs to a larger family of viruses called *Orthomyxoviridae*. Each of the three influenza viruses has distinct characteristics, including the following:

- organization of the genetic material contained within the virus
- viral structure
- preference of the viral strain for a certain type of host
- certain epidemiological associations
- symptoms exhibited by infected patients

However, there are some similarities between the A, B, and C influenza viruses, including their surrounding envelope and the type of genetic material, or genome, contained within it.

The diameter of an influenza virus is approximately 80 to 120 nanometers. Thus, influenza can best be seen with the assistance of an electron microscope (see Figure 1.4). The influenza virus can exist either in the form of a sphere or as elongated filamentous particles and requires travel in air droplets because of its enveloped structure. As aerosolized droplets are inhaled by a host, viral particles contaminate the mucosal layer of the respiratory tract, penetrate the mucus, and enter a host cell to begin replication.

Influenza viruses have a genome composed of single-stranded RNA in eight separate segments. This RNA encodes genes for eight different proteins.

Overlying the structural matrix is a fatty bilayer membrane called an envelope, which actually is derived from the host cell that produced the viral particle. The envelope is covered with projections or spikes; these are glycoproteins. In the case of influenza A, the spikes contain either hemagglutinin (HA) or neuraminidase (NA), along with the membrane protein M2. At least sixteen different HAs have been described (H1 to H16), whereas at least nine different NAs have been identified (N1 to N9). These proteins have allowed scientists to classify strains of influenza in different species of mammals and to determine their likelihood of causing infection in humans. The type of HA and NA proteins exhibited by a specific influenza strain is of major significance, because it influences virulence and becomes very important in attempts to predict, prevent, control, or treat outbreaks of the disease. Naming an influenza virus isolate also involves identification of HA and NA proteins. Full nomenclature first requires the influenza virus type (usually A or B), host species (left out if human), geographical site, serial number, year of isolation, and, finally, HA and NA variants in parentheses. Thus, a fully identified avian influenza isolate may read "A/goose/Guangdong/1/96 (H5N1)." Despite all of the possible

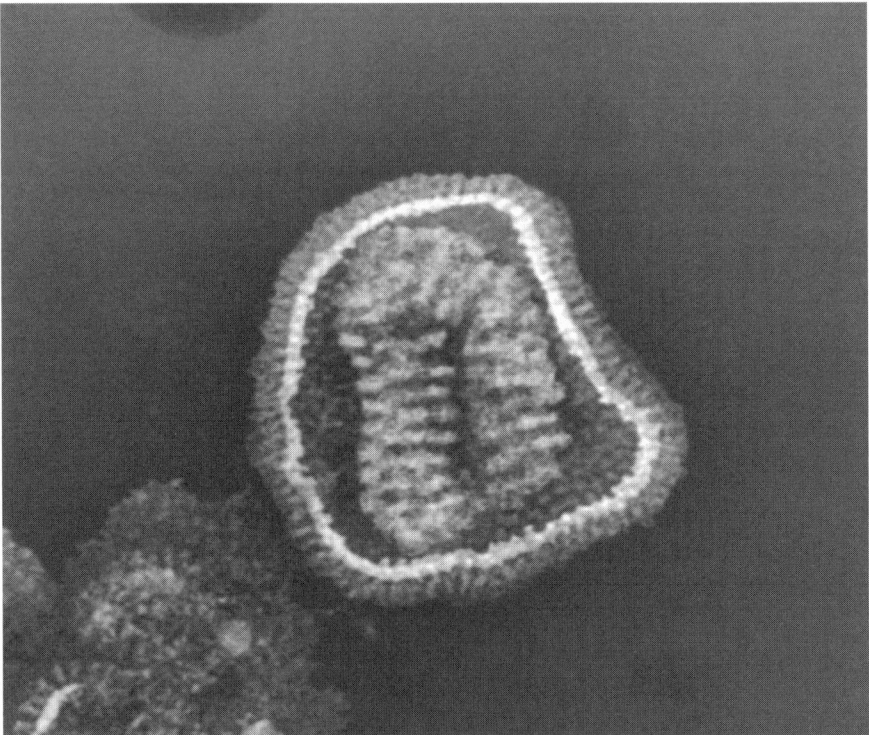

Figure 1.4. Electron Micrograph of Influenza A. Negative-stained transmission electron micrograph depicting the ultrastructural details of an influenza virus particle, or virion. Image credited to Cynthia Goldsmith; used with permission, courtesy of the CDC.

combinations of HA and NA antigens, only two strains have, in recent history, been found in circulation within the human population as the cause of seasonal outbreaks: H1N1 and H3N2. The occurrence of a new strain of influenza with either unrecognized HA and NA antigens is a major concern.

Both HA and NA have very specific functions. HA is so named because it allows red blood cells (which contain hemoglobin) to clump, or agglutinate. The main portion of the HA protein projects outward from the viral envelope like a spike, allowing at least five different recognizable, antigenic sites to be presented. Once the viral particle has entered the respiratory tract of a host, it is the function of HA to allow attachment of the virus to the receptors on the surface of the human cell. Specifically, HA binds to sialic acid found on the surface of the cells in a process called adsorption. The influenza virus then enters the cell through the membrane, protected by a bubble called a vesicle. If the virus cannot penetrate the particular cell it initially targets, it will detach and

Proteins Encoded by Influenza RNA

Polymerase B2 protein (PB2), polymerase B1 protein (PB1), and polymerase A protein (PA): Forms an active RNA-RNA bond, which is ultimately responsible for viral replication and transcription.

Nucleocapsid protein (NP): Links to the RNA-RNA bond.

Matrix protein (M1): Forms a structural matrix surrounding the genetic material.

Matrix protein (M2): Acts as an ion channel pump with a goal of pH (acid-base) adjustment.

Nonstructural proteins (NS): Regulates the synthesis of viral components in an infected cell.

Hemagglutinin (HA): Allows attachment of the virus to the receptors on the surface of the human cell.

Neuraminidase (NA): Enables a newly created virion to separate from the host cell.

move on to bind to another cell to try again. Once inside a cell, the virion (and HA spike) undergoes a shift in position, which allows the shedding of the viral coat. The viral genes then spill into the cell, and penetration of the viral RNA strands into the host cell's nucleus occurs. Once there, the virion uses the host cell's machinery to process proteins. These are packaged into new viral particles, which are then free to leave the host cell and travel along the respiratory tract to find new cells to target for infection. Amazingly, it takes only six to ten hours for the entire replication process to occur.

NA also presents most of its structure to the outside of the lipid membrane layer, and it is an important antigenic site. Its presence appears to be necessary for full penetration of the virion through the host's mucus layer, which lines the respiratory tract. Perhaps more importantly, however, NA has an enzymatic function, which enables a newly created virion to separate from the host cell and travel freely from one cell to another through the respiratory tract, and, ultimately, out of the respiratory tract to a new victim. NA accomplishes this function specifically by cleaving sialic acid receptor from the HA molecule, from other NA proteins, and from glycoproteins and glycolipids at the host cell surface. If NA did not allow HA cleavage, the new viral particles could bind to the sialic acid receptors on the cell surface as they attempt to travel, and their chance of infecting new cells would be diminished. During the replication process, thousands upon thousands of new influenza viral particles can be produced and released.

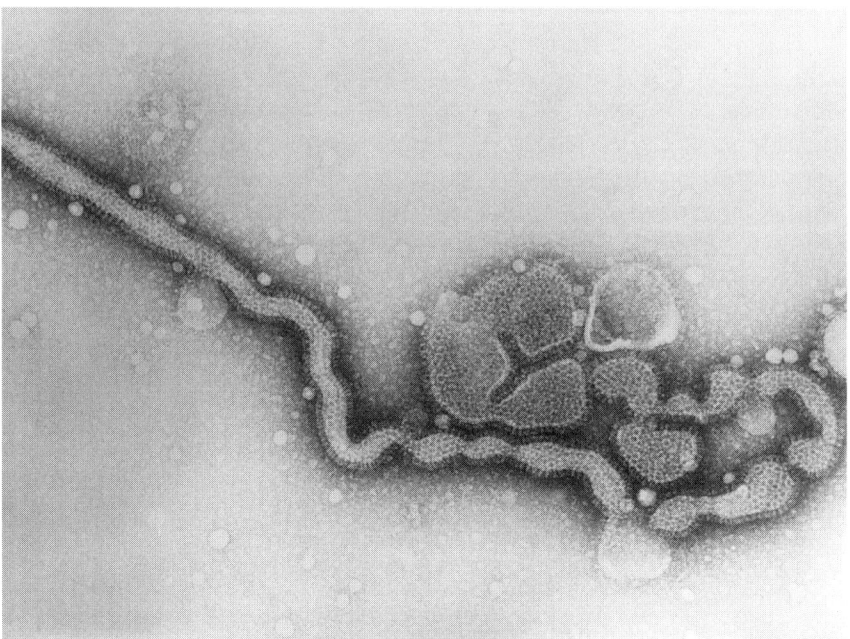

Figure 1.5. Electron Micrograph of Influenza C. A transmission electron micrograph depicting the variable morphology of an influenza C viral strain. Image used with permission, courtesy of the CDC.

The influenza C virus differs from A and B in that it has only seven genome segments, and its surface carries only one glycoprotein (see Figure 1.5). Because this virus has little to do with human disease, it will not be discussed further here.

VIRAL PATHOGENICITY AND HOST RESPONSES

To be successful, an infectious agent needs to be able to travel from host to host to perpetuate its disease process, without actually interrupting its transmission by causing death of the host. Influenza, obviously, is a nearly perfect virus in this respect. It can infect millions of hosts during an outbreak and has managed to survive as a pathogen for humans (and other living creatures) for centuries. How, then, does influenza manage to be so efficacious, and what response does the human host mount against it? The pathogenicity and virulence of influenza are attributable to factors intrinsic to the virus itself as well as to factors inherent in the human host.

Viral Factors

As already discussed, the influenza virus has specific antigenic sites on its glyco-protein spikes that allow recognition by host cells and eventual penetration into the cell to facilitate viral replication. The proteins encoded by the virus sequester viral RNA, attempting to prevent recognition by the host cell and, hopefully, stalling detection by the immune system and eventual interferon release. During the replication process, the virus kills the host cell by a number of different mechanisms: (1) shutting down the host cell's ability to make its own proteins, (2) degrading the cell's genetic messenger material, (3) blocking genetic transcription of the infected cell, (4) allowing further breakdown of cellular proteins, and (5) causing damage to the cell's DNA. While the cell is dying, the newly replicated viral particles are released. This entire process takes time, and, usually, eighteen to seventy-two hours pass between acquisition of the virus and the onset of identifiable symptoms in the host; this is known as the incubation period.

There are many factors that may account for the ability of influenza viruses to infect their hosts and make them ill but still allow transmission of viral particles to new hosts. One essential feature has been shown to be the cleavage of the HA. This concept is important, because some of the current strains of avian flu are not likely to cause human disease as a result of inadequate HA cleavage.

Another mechanism that allows spread of the influenza infection from host to host is known as viral shedding. During the incubation period, virus can be detected in the respiratory secretions of infected patients before any onset of identifiable symptoms. The number of viral particles increases to a peak fairly rapidly thereafter, remains elevated for twenty-four to forty-eight hours, and then rapidly decreases to low levels. Usually, an infected patient can shed virus for five to ten days, although children and immune-compromised patients appear to shed virus for longer periods of time. The severity of systemic symptoms seems to correlate with the quantity of virus shed in sick individuals.

In addition to the viral factors that contribute to successful infection within a host, the influenza virus is notorious for its ability to undergo antigenic variation and recombination from zoonotic sources. It is this tendency for mutation that prevents lifelong immunity against influenza in the human population and leads to the increasing concern for a future pandemic that might mimic the morbidity and mortality of the 1918 outbreak.

Host Factors

The human body has a defense system that stands ready to defend the host against invasion by an unwelcome pathogen. Even as an infectious agent enters the respiratory tract of a new host, the victim attempts to limit its chance of harmful infection. Saliva itself contains enzymes that attempt to destroy pathogens. Hairs in the nose provide an obstacle that might hinder the travels of a large pathogen. Mucus is secreted along the lining of the respiratory tract, trapping debris and organisms and encouraging its travel back up the throat to be swallowed. The respiratory epithelial cells directly underneath the mucus layer have projections called cilia, which continuously beat in a sweeping motion, trying to move unwanted pathogens so they can be expelled. The acts of coughing and sneezing force fluid, mucus, and, hopefully, the offending pathogens outward. The influenza virus is thus dispersed in aerosols (each containing large volumes of virions) from the respiratory tract of a sick patient.

Once the virus has successfully navigated the physical defenses of its new host, it must attach to and penetrate the cells lining the respiratory tract to begin replication. It is fortunate for the virus, then, that human respiratory epithelial cells actually have receptors on their surface that recognize and receive the pathogen. It is also to the virus' benefit that enzymes in the host cell are available to assist with entry into the cell and the subsequent initiation of replication.

When infected with the influenza virus, the human host has a clear and identifiable immune response, and the degree of illness is dependent on both the host's state of immune competence and any specific immunity that may have developed in response to previous viral infection. The immune system defense is coordinated and complicated and includes both antibody production (known as humoral immunity) and cytoxic white blood cell responses (known as cellular immunity).

Antibodies are proteins that are produced by plasma cells in response to exposure to specific sites (known as antigens) on the surface of an infectious pathogen. Antibodies infer long-lived resistance to reinfection with the same antigen because, once activated, plasma cells can differentiate into memory cells that will produce new antibodies when infection is again recognized. Thus, hosts that survive an acute viral infection are, for the most part, immune to infections by the same virus. Unfortunately, this concept does not hold true in the case of influenza. Because of the virus' tendency to mutate, or shift, humans are unable to elicit an immune response that would prevent infection with all subtypes or strains of the virus.

In response to initial infection with the influenza virus, antibody formation against the HA and NA glycoproteins, as well as to the membrane and nucleocapsid proteins, occurs in the host, both system wide and locally within the respiratory tract itself. Antibodies produced against HA actually neutralize the influenza virus and reduce its ability to infect other cells. The antibody against NA, on the other hand, reduces the release of virus from already infected cells; this decreases the severity of host symptoms while also limiting viral shedding. Antibodies manufactured to target membrane and nucleocapsid proteins do not appear to render the virus ineffective, and they do not play a role in protective immunity against future infections, either. These antibodies do, however, provide a marker that can be measured in the bloodstream of infected patients and thus can be useful for diagnosis of recent infection. Peak antibody production is measurable about four to seven weeks after infection, and the levels decline slowly thereafter; however, low levels of antibodies can often be detected years after infection.

In addition to antibody production, the host has a cellular immune response. Activated T-lymphocytes (a type of white blood cell) migrate to the site of infection to mediate antiviral activities: CD8 T-lymphocytes help kill host cells that have been invaded by virus, whereas CD4 T-lymphocytes help with generation of antibodies and activation of cells that produce cytokines. Both infected epithelial cells and immune cells of the respiratory mucosa release cytokines, which include interferon, tumor necrosis factor, and interleukins. These hormones have multiple functions, including initiation of an inflammatory cascade, which can cause redness, heat, and swelling at the site of infection and systemically throughout the body; thus, it is the cytokine response that is the cause of fever during infection with influenza. Interferon forces cells to make a variety of proteins in an attempt to thwart the virus. The most important of these proteins is a type of phosphokinase, which prevents viruses from using RNA for replication. Tumor necrosis factor, conversely, is a toxin and can be lethal to cells.

Although the inflammatory reaction triggered by the cytokine release and the upregulation of the immune system is meant to be protective to the infected host, it can also cause great harm. At a cellular level, tumor necrosis factor, released in an attempt to destroy infected cells, can prove deadly to nearby healthy cells as well. Immune cells known as macrophages can release a substance that upregulates the bone marrow and promotes production of more white blood cells that act as the body's defense; unfortunately, activity within the marrow can cause severe pain in the bones. Epithelial cells lining the respiratory tract are killed in great numbers, leaving the upper tract bare and the throat raw. While the immune system focuses on eradicating the virus, the body's defenses against bacteria are lessened, and secondary infection can occur. Mucus and fluid produced along the respiratory tract in response to infection can clog the airways. If the lower respiratory tract becomes involved in the infection, capillaries can be obliterated, and bleeding or hemorrhaging can result. Debris from dying cells and old blood collects along the respiratory tract, and the lung cells produce a protective fibrin-like connective tissue to aid in healing; these substances can disrupt the transfer of oxygen between blood and the lung's air sacs, and, eventually, the lung tissue begins to die. Finally, a clinical condition known as adult respiratory distress syndrome (ARDS) can occur. ARDS essentially represents disintegration of lung tissue, leaving a patient with a 50:50 chance of survival, even with intensive medical care.

It has become clear that the cytokine response and the resulting inflammatory cascade may differ depending on the infecting influenza viral strain. A strain identified in 1997, called Hong Kong H5N1, has been suggested to potently induce cytokine release, and this may account for its excessive lethality. In fatal cases of infection with this strain, manifestations beyond ARDS have been described, including necrosis of liver cells, kidney damage, and depletion of white blood cells. It is also possible that a vigorous inflammatory response triggered by infection of patients in 1918 was, in part, responsible for the quick and painful deaths of some of its victims, resulting in the skewed mortality curves featuring predominately young adults during that pandemic. Additional details regarding the H5N1 influenza strain can be found in Chapter 2, and the influenza pandemic of 1918 is discussed at great length in Chapter 3.

2

The Epidemiology of Influenza

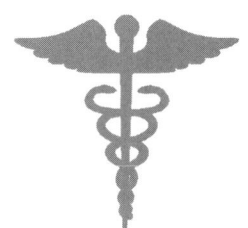

It is perfectly obvious that no one nor any single country can save the world from the horrors of tsunamis, hurricanes, earthquakes, and winged influenza.

Richard Reeves, Presidential Scholar
and Award-Winning Political Filmmaker, 2005

DEFINITIONS AND TIMELINES

In 1918, a strain of influenza known as the Spanish Flu raced across the world, infecting and killing millions of people. Although few people today remember the pandemic or recall even learning about the event in school, some scientists have studied influenza with intensity and can now distinctly outline its path through time. The timeline found in this book provides a sense of influenza's history and important clinical and research milestones, but it only hints at the importance the virus' epidemiology holds for studies in the future. Although the 1918 pandemic is considered a part of the world's collective history now, influenza continues to have significant impact as a disease, with impressive global consequences. In its seasonal outbreaks, it can affect 10–20 percent of the total world population. Annual epidemics in developed countries are thought to result in 3–5 million cases of severe illness and 250,000–500,000 deaths each year. Data from the tropical and developing countries are limited with regard to accurate reporting, but the disease is known to have high attack rates and can cause considerable morbidity and mortality in these parts of the world. Thus, the study of the influenza, and the virus that causes it, continues with great interest.

In considering influenza, it is important to understand the terminology used to describe its disease manifestations with regard to populations. An outbreak refers to the occurrence of a large number of cases of a disease in a short period of time. Outbreaks of influenza are common and occur yearly in many places. An epidemic refers to an outbreak that is confined to one location, such as a city or a country. Unfortunately, epidemics remain somewhat unpredictable with regard to the timing of onset and the severity of illness. Certain features make influenza epidemics more likely, including the following:

1. winter months attributable to cold weather, crowding of people (usually to escape the cold), and high humidity
2. origination of the outbreak in either Eastern or Southern Hemisphere countries, with later spread to Europe and North America
3. occurrence of a variant virus with antigenic changes from previously recognized strains (this concept will be discussed in more detail later in this chapter)
4. presence of human cross-reacting antibody, acquired during previous infection, is low in the population, with regard to both the percentage of people positive for the antibody and the level of antibody present in positive individuals

During a typical influenza epidemic, attack rates are estimated to be 10–20 percent, but, in certain populations, it can reach 40–50 percent. In temperate climates, epidemics tend to occur almost exclusively in winter months (October to April in the Northern Hemisphere and May to September in the Southern Hemisphere). Isolated cases, or even outbreaks, of influenza A have been reported during the warm weather months. In the tropics, influenza can be seen year round. Summertime epidemics of influenza have occurred on cruise ships in both the Northern and Southern Hemispheres. Airline travel has also been linked to influenza outbreaks.

In most epidemics, a single strain of influenza will dominate, and other respiratory viruses decrease in frequency. Influenza A epidemics typically begin rather abruptly, peak over a two- to three-week period, and then last for two to three months in total. Usually, children are the first to suffer (often with an illness characterized by fever and respiratory symptoms). Increases in adult infections (with typical flu-like symptoms) soon follow. Later manifestations of epidemics include absenteeism from school and work. Influenza B epidemics are generally less extensive and are associated with milder disease than those caused by influenza A. Often, the outbreaks of influenza B are reported in schools, military camps, chronic-care facilities, and nursing homes; it has also caused at least one identified outbreak on a cruise ship.

On occasion, two different strains of influenza circulate simultaneously. In addition, epidemics of influenza may occur during outbreaks of other respiratory viruses, such as adenovirus or respiratory syncytial virus. In some years, the end of an influenza epidemic is characterized by a brief spike in cases attributable to an entirely new strain of influenza. These mini-outbreaks are known as a "herald wave," and they give scientists a clue as to the likely dominant strain of the flu for the next season.

For an outbreak to be labeled a pandemic, several conditions must be satisfied: (1) after arising in a specific geographical area, the outbreak of infection spreads throughout the world; (2) a high percentage of individuals are infected, which then results in an increased death rate; and (3) the infection is caused by a new influenza A serotype, which is not related to the viruses that circulated immediately before and did not arise via mutation of the preceding viruses. Some characteristics of pandemics include the following:

- extremely rapid transmission with concurrent outbreaks throughout the globe
- the occurrence of disease outside the usual seasonality (including summer months)
- high attack rates in all age groups, with increased risk for complications and death in healthy young adults not generally affected by seasonal influenza
- more severe symptoms in affected populations
- high likelihood of increased mortality rates
- multiple waves of disease immediately before and after the main outbreak

There are ongoing arguments in the medical and historical literature regarding the number of pandemics that have actually occurred as a result of influenza. Most references agree that there have been at least three in the last century.

The descriptions of the previous influenza pandemics are oftentimes disturbing, but understanding them to the fullest extent possible is necessary if

Influenza Pandemics of the Twentieth Century

The Spanish Flu, 1918: It was the most lethal outbreak of influenza ever and killed an estimated 20-50 million people worldwide. The spread of the virus was facilitated by the movement of troops involved in World War I. Second and third waves of infection occurred, with the latter waves being more deadly than the first. The influenza strain was ultimately identified as H1N1. (This pandemic will be discussed in great detail in Chapter 3, because it remains the standard against which all other modern pandemics are measured.)

The Asian Flu, 1957: This pandemic started in the Yunan Province of China in February. After causing many to become ill in China during March, it spread to Hong Kong, Singapore, Taiwan, and then Japan. Infection spread to India, Australia, and Indonesia in May; to Pakistan, Europe, North America, and the Middle East in June; to South Africa, South America, New Zealand, and the Pacific Islands in July; and to Central, West, and East Africa, eastern Europe, and the Caribbean in August. Interestingly, a large conference held in Iowa served as a major landline for infection. Eighteen hundred young adults from forty-three states and several foreign countries attended the conference; 200 of the attendees fell ill with influenza. These individuals then returned home and facilitated spread of the infection elsewhere. Another landline was identified from Russia to Scandinavia and Eastern Europe; otherwise, the infection appears to have spread by sea travel. Within six months, the infection was worldwide. A second wave of infection occurred in early 1958, with regions in Europe, North America, Russia, and Japan involved. In some countries, the second wave was more severe. In total, the pandemic affected 40–50% of the world's population, with 25–30% showing signs or symptoms of the disease. The mortality rate was estimated to be 1 in 4,000; most deaths were in the very young and the very old. The strain was identified as H2N2, a subtype never before seen in the human population.

The Hong Kong Flu, 1968: This pandemic killed thousands of people worldwide (estimates suggest 700,000–1,000,000), including 34,000 in the United States. It began in Hong Kong in the summer months, traveled to Vietnam and Singapore, and eventually on to India, the Philippines, Australia, and Europe. The virus traveled to the United States in September but peaked in December and January of 1969 with regard to mortality. Additional waves in 1969 and 1970 were also deadly and included cases in Japan, Africa, and South America. The decreased death rate compared with previous pandemics was thought to be multifactorial: possible partial immunity attributable to similarities to the 1957 Asian Flu strain, better medical care, and availability of antibiotics to combat secondary bacterial infections. The strain was identified as H3N2, a virus subtype still in circulation today.

preparation for a future pandemic is to be adequate. In addition to the great numbers of illnesses and deaths caused by influenza across the globe, the pandemics have had devastating consequences on social and economic circumstances in many countries. Experts agree that another influenza pandemic is inevitable and possibly imminent. In 2003, a WHO Report by the Secretariat on Influenza projected that, if a new pandemic occurs, it will result, in industrialized countries alone, in 57–132 million outpatient healthcare visits, 1.0–2.3 million hospital admissions, and 280,000–650,000 deaths in less than two years. In developing countries, the impact is likely to be even more substantial. More recent estimates suggest that the appearance of a pandemic influenza virus could cause close to 3 million deaths in the United States and more than 100 million deaths worldwide. In addition to such startling statistics, other issues come to mind when considering a future pandemic, namely, the inability of healthcare systems to meet the demands cast on them during such an outbreak (for instance, there will likely be shortages of medical personnel, lack of respirators for all needy patients, inadequate isolation wards to limit spread of the disease, and too few hospital beds and other equipment for the numbers afflicted by the disease) and the worry that treatment will be delayed enough to clearly affect the death rates (for example, vaccines may be unavailable in the early phase of a pandemic, with concurrent shortages of effective antiviral drugs in early weeks and months of the outbreak). Additional discussion of pandemic concerns and measures for future preparation can be found in Chapter 3.

INFLUENZA ANTIGENIC DRIFT AND SHIFT

The influenza virus is decidedly skillful in its ability to alter its surface proteins. As previously discussed, glycoprotein spikes on the viral surface have been identified as HA and NA. Using HA and NA, the influenza virus is able to infect a host cell to undergo protein synthesis and, ultimately, to succeed with viral replication. However, the genes for encoding the HA and NA proteins of influenza are found along an RNA, rather than DNA, backbone. DNA-based viruses have a special proofreading enzyme that carefully scrutinizes the process of copying a strand of DNA, catching and correcting any mistakes made during replication. Unfortunately, RNA-based viruses like influenza do not have a proofreader. During replication of the virus, mistakes occur, particularly with regard to the HA and NA molecules. The mutation of antigenic sites, or points on the HA and NA molecules where antibodies would normally bind, is known as antigenic drift. The influenza virus mutates so quickly that 99 percent of the new viral particles produced in a host cell are defective. Most of the mutations cause defects that are severe enough to either destroy the new virion completely or hinder its ability to infect a new cell. Other mutations, however, allow the new viral particle to adapt to its new situation, potentially producing a more dangerous infectious agent. Most of these mutations are thought to be point mutations in the RNA gene segments that code for the HA or the NA proteins, or the exchange of one amino acid for another.

When HA and NA molecules are changed, it affects the ability of a human host's protective antibodies to bind to their sites and to trigger an immune response to infection. With progression of antigenic drift, a decline in protective antibodies acquired during infection in earlier years occurs. Humans become less able to defend themselves against a constantly mutating virus because their old antibodies may not recognize a newly changed strain or they may not work as well (if recognition is accomplished at all). This explains, then, the repeated pattern of influenza epidemics for centuries on end. Scientists and public health experts monitor the antigenic drift of influenza carefully, and the influenza vaccine produced each year attempts to take into consideration the possible mutations that might have influenced the next season's strain(s) of virus.

The influenza subtypes that cause pandemic influenza do not arise by mutation from existing strains; thus, the origin of these viruses remains the focus of much research. The most accepted theory suggests that pandemic viruses arise from a cross of avian and human strains with drastic alterations in the viral HA and NA structures, a phenomenon known as antigenic shift. In this process, an avian influenza virus and a human influenza virus initiate a "double infection" in a cell of a species in which they can both multiply (such as the pig). While replicating, the virus undergoes reassortment with genetic material from each strain, allowing infectivity in humans, but with the presence of an avian HA glycoprotein to which the majority of the human population has never been exposed (and thus has no antibodies). If two different viruses infect a cell, an exchange of gene segments can easily take place, with the mathematical consequence of hundreds of different "offspring." The offspring viral particles, then, have the potential to infect many humans with no hope of immunity and to cause severe disease and even death. With sixteen different HA and nine distinct NA subtypes, new influenza offspring can be named according to their particular variation in HA and NA molecules. For example, the influenza virus found to have been the culprit in the 1918 pandemic was H1N1, and a cause of the 1976 swine flu scare (see Chapter 6 for more details) was also H1N1. The bird flu scare of 1997, however, was caused by the presence of H5N1, a viral strain that had never before been seen in humans.

SIGNIFICANCE OF INFLUENZA STRAIN H5N1

In 1997, the identification of the avian influenza strain H5N1 in Hong Kong caused great concern within the medical and public health communities (see Figure 2.1). With the assistance of WHO, an immediate investigation was initiated. With poor sanitation an issue at poultry farms and at the live poultry markets in Hong Kong, the avian H5N1 influenza strain is thought to have spread directly from chickens to humans. During the twelve months of 1997, it infected eighteen people, and all of those who became ill with H5N1 had massive exposure to the virus attributable to handling of poultry. The morbidity and mortality associated with this influenza strain were impressive: more than 60 percent of the infected suffered from severe pneumonia, and 51 percent required treatment in an intensive care unit. Ultimately, six of the eighteen infected humans died, resulting in a mortality rate of 33 percent. Autopsy analysis of two of the victims revealed unusually high levels of cytokines

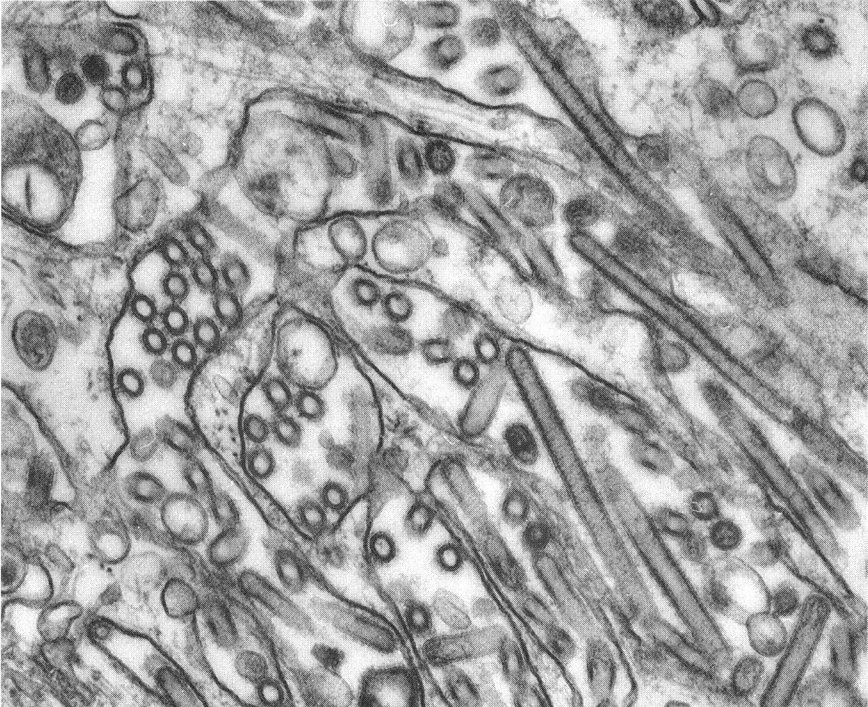

Figure 2.1. Electron Micrograph of Avian Influenza H5N1. Transmission electron micrograph of avian influenza A, strain H5N1, in both rounded and filamentous forms. Image credited to Cynthia Goldsmith; used with permission, courtesy of the CDC.

(interferon and tumor necrosis factor). As was discussed in Chapter 1, cytokines are substances released in response to infection that regulate the intensity and duration of the immune response. The vigorous response of cytokines, while attempting to eliminate the unwanted pathogen, unfortunately caused consequences that, in conjunction with the viral infection, were fatally harmful to the host.

In response to the H5N1 outbreak, the entire poultry population (consisting of more than 1 million chickens) in China was destroyed within three days. Despite this, circulation of H5N1 has continued, and the number of human cases continues to rise. The timeline included in this book gives a sense of the spread of this viral strain. To date, more than 350 cases have been identified in humans.

Although the 1997 outbreak was a direct consequence of exposure to chickens for its victims, a mutation in the virus occurred that allowed it to bind to a human cell's sialic acid receptor. Usually, an influenza virus that binds to a bird's sialic acid receptor cannot bind to the receptor in humans, thus preventing infection from avian influenza in the human host. Luckily, during the 1997 outbreak, the mutation did not allow human-to-human transmission, and the behaviors thought responsible for transmission included handling, plucking, and preparing diseased birds, and consumption of ducks' blood or undercooked poultry.

In 2003, H5N1 was again found in humans. Two members of a family returning from mainland China to Hong Kong had confirmed cases of influenza caused by H5N1; a third relative died of a respiratory illness, but the diagnosis of influenza was never established. Although small in number, the finding of the virus among family members has raised concern for human-to-human spread; fortunately, this method of transmission appears to be limited and, as of yet, has not caused a sustained outbreak.

However, the concept of human-to-human transmission of a novel, avian influenza is exactly what causes concern for a future pandemic. As has been suggested earlier in this chapter, there are certain prerequisites that are required for a pandemic: (1) a new viral subtype must emerge to which humans have little or no immunity, (2) the new virus must be able to replicate in humans and cause disease, and (3) the new virus must be able to be efficiently transmitted from one human to another. With the H5N1 strain, the first two criteria have already been met. Although it is not certain whether H5N1 will undergo additional mutations, it may only be a matter of time before the third prerequisite is fulfilled. In that case, pandemic influenza may be unavoidable.

Some new developments with the H5N1 influenza strain have now been identified and add to the global worry of an inevitable pandemic:

- Since the initial outbreak of H5N1 in 1997, documented human infections have been confirmed in Thailand, Vietnam, Indonesia, Cambodia, China, Turkey, Azerbaijan, Laos, Djibouti, Egypt, Nigeria, Iraq, Pakistan, and Myanmar. Over 350 human cases have been identified, and the overall lethality has exceeded 60 percent.
- Although the majority of human cases have been characterized predominantly by respiratory manifestations, there is evidence of extrapulmonary disease in some victims. In one patient who suffered from encephalopathy and diarrhea, the H5N1 virus was isolated from cerebrospinal fluid and from rectal swab specimens.
- The H5N1 infections documented in some aquatic birds, including swans and geese, have been severe with regard to the clinical manifestations of the avian host; this is unusual, because influenza has traditionally been an asymptomatic infection for birds.
- Viral shedding has been documented from the gastrointestinal tract of the aquatic birds (as would be expected) but now also from the respiratory tract. In animal models of H5N1 infection, the virus has been found in nervous, urinary, gastrointestinal, and lymphoid tissue.
- Felines have been infected with H5N1 strains of influenza, a highly unusual occurrence. Domestic cats have died as a result of infection with the virus, and infection in felines has been reproduced in the laboratory setting. In Thailand, two tigers and two leopards at the Bangkok Zoo were infected with the H5N1 virus after eating raw chicken carcasses; the cats all died with fever and respiratory difficulties. Other felines who had not been fed the raw chicken carcasses also became ill, suggesting horizontal transmission of the virus from cat to cat.
- A fatal case of avian H5N1 influenza has also been reported in a dog.
- A mutation involving the M2 protein in the H5N1 strain has conferred resistance to the antiviral medications amantadine and rimantadine, known as M2 inhibitors. Two mechanisms of resistance against neuraminidase inhibitors (oseltamivir and zanamivir) have been described that involve mutations in either the NA or the HA gene.

Significant surveillance measures are in place, both in the United States and across the globe, to track the activity of avian influenza viral strains and to monitor the virus' mutations and resulting resistance patterns. Additional detail regarding the national and worldwide pandemic preparation measures currently in place can be found in Chapter 3.

Additional Avian Influenza Strains

In addition to H5N1, several other avian influenza viruses have been linked to human disease in recent years:

- A strain identified as H10N7 has been reported for the first time in humans with illness in two infants in Egypt. One child's father is a poultry worker.
- An avian strain H9N2 has been isolated in children from Hong Kong; all had mild and short-lived respiratory infections. Because genes found in the H9N2 strain appear to be homologous to H5N1 genes, it is thought that reassortment occurred between the two viruses. H9N2 is still in circulation and is considered endemic in poultry and bird markets in Asia and has also been isolated from pigs.
- In 2003, extensive outbreaks of H7N7 avian influenza virus occurred in poultry in The Netherlands. Workers who were responsible for controlling this outbreak became ill: eighty-one suffered from conjunctivitis alone, two had a flu-like illness along with conjunctivitis, and two had isolated respiratory symptoms. Human-to-human transmission was documented in three household contacts. One veterinarian developed a fatal respiratory infection; his strain of H7N7 was found to have a number of mutations when compared with the strain causing conjunctivitis.
- A strain identified as H7N3 has been reported for the first time in humans with a conjunctival illness occurring in two poultry workers in Canada.
- A strain identified as H7N2 has caused hospitalization of a patient in New York, and United Kingdom Health Protection has reported at least four human infections with a low pathogenic avian influenza strain of H7N2. The cases were associated with concurrent poultry infection.

3

The Influenza Pandemic of 1918

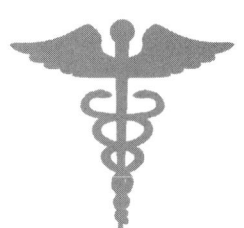

Well, certainly we can say that there will be new pandemics. That's certainly the history of influenza viruses. And it's—it's possible that there would be a pandemic of this magnitude. One could hope that there wouldn't be, but I think we should be prepared for that possibility.

Dr. Jeffrey Taubenberger,
Chief of the Division of Molecular Pathology,
Armed Forces Institute of Pathology, 2005

The influenza pandemic of 1918 may be the most dramatic and devastating medical event that has ever occurred in history. Previously written descriptions of the pandemic attempt to convey the enormity of its consequences by noting that it was "the greatest medical holocaust in history" (Waring, 1971, p. 33). In the United States alone, one of every four people suffered from the effects of the virus, and more than 500,000 deaths were recorded. Worldwide, an estimated 20–50 million people died during the pandemic (although, by some estimates, the number may be as high as 100 million). Amazingly, this influenza pandemic was actually responsible for more deaths than all of the major wars of the twentieth century combined. And, in contrast to other outbreaks of influenza, the great majority of deaths during the pandemic occurred in previously healthy young adults. Indeed, the impact was so significant that the life expectancy in the United States dropped by more than ten years in 1918.

DESCRIPTION OF THE PANDEMIC

Despite such atrocities, it has only been in recent history that the 1918 influenza pandemic has garnered much attention with either the greater medical community or the general public. And now, more than ever, an understanding of the events of that outbreak is necessary if humankind is to attempt to survive, or perhaps even prevent, another such pandemic.

In 1918, the world was already engaged in World War I, which had started in 1914. The United States entered the war in April of 1917. In March of 1918, almost a year after President Woodrow Wilson agreed to enter the war, nearly 100,000 American troops were sent to Europe; the following month, almost 120,000 made the trip. While the soldiers battled forces in Europe, folks left behind in the States were suffering from springtime influenza. Soldiers remaining at base camps across the United States asked for treatments to relieve fever, headache, backache, and malaise. Workers at the Ford Motor Company in Detroit were sent home because of illness. Prisoners at the San Quentin Prison in California were diagnosed with the flu. Some of those afflicted with influenza in March, April, and May had fairly severe cases, and some were also diagnosed with pneumonia. The infection rate in North America was quite high, but it did not appear that this would be a particularly virulent outbreak, because deaths were not excessively appreciated at the time.

The exact origin of the first wave of the 1918 pandemic is still not known. Although some literature suggests that it may have originated in China, other documentation describes several of the first outbreaks as those in Detroit, Kansas, South Carolina, and San Quentin Prison. From these focal points in the United States, the infection could easily have spread outward and then eastward. As American troops were sent to Europe to various army and naval training sites in preparation for war, influenza went with them. Traveling by ship, influenza was passed from the North American military personnel to soldiers at the Bordeaux, France, depot in mid-April of 1918. From France, the virus then spread to the British Expeditionary Force and to other European soldiers involved in the war. By late April and May, the infection had also reached Italy and Spain. Outbreaks in Germany began to be described as well.

In June, the disease reached England, Scotland, and Wales. It made its way quickly through the military, with cases in the British Army exceeding 30,000 during June, more than six times the number reported in May. Influenza struck Portugal and then Greece. It moved to Murmansk via the British troops and eventually arrived in Russia. From this point, the illness spread quickly to North Africa, Bombay, and Calcutta and then on to China, New Zealand, and the Philippines.

The flu was quite impressively contagious as it traveled the globe. In some military regiments, 90 percent of soldiers became infected with the virus. The disease began to be known as the Spanish Influenza, despite the fact that it certainly did not originate in Spain. Spain, instead, was a neutral country during the war and did not have government censorship of its press. Thus, whereas French, German, and British newspapers were not allowed to print anything negative that might hurt morale, the Spanish papers honestly reported the presence of influenza, including the affliction of King Alphonse XIII with the virus. Spain was one of the few countries to openly report the presence of the disease and its effect on both its troops and its civilians.

Early on, there was not much to suggest that this pandemic would be particularly exceptional: other pandemics had followed a similar rate of spread, and the number of deaths was thought to be comparable with past outbreaks. In July of 1918, some physicians from England concluded that the epidemic was not even attributable to influenza, because the symptoms for most patients were mild, the illness did not appear to last long, and most cases were not likely to relapse or to progress to complications. Unfortunately, it also escaped the world's attention that most of the deaths attributable to the spring wave of influenza had occurred in healthy young adults. Later review of historical documentation, including analysis of death claims made in 1918 against the Metropolitan Life Insurance Company in the United States, would reveal that a small, but unexpected, number of infected patients died of the disease during the spring wave of illness, and that most of those deaths occurred in young people aged twenty-one to twenty-nine. Perhaps this trend was overlooked as a result of the concurrent number of deaths occurring in young adults because of the war. As influenza made its way across continents, young soldiers were engaged in deadly military combat, and many young men perished during battle. Alongside the war injuries and deaths, the influenza virus caused its own military devastation: troops were weakened by illness, and some offensives launched in the spring and summer of 1918 by Germany's soldiers were thought to have failed in part because of poor morale and diminished strength of the armies attributable to the flu.

In most every country during the first wave of influenza in 1918, the infection spread for several weeks and then faded sharply. Although ships would continue to arrive at American ports as the weather turned warm and passengers and crew suffered from influenza during their voyages, only an occasional, isolated outbreak was diagnosed during the summer of 1918 in the United

States. It was suggested that perhaps being exposed to influenza during the spring wave of infection granted Americans protection during the summer, a concept known as "herd immunity." In mid-August, the British command actually declared the influenza epidemic over.

Unfortunately, despite leaving U.S. soil as healthy soldiers, many young men traveled to Europe in June, July, and August for war, just as the Europeans were experiencing a severe second wave of infection with influenza. During those three months, more than half a million troops made the trip from the United States to Europe. Although the risk of such transport during a time of European disease outbreak was recognized, the movement was not interrupted. As Colonel S. M. Kennedy, chief surgeon of the New York Port of Embarkation, said, "[W]e can't stop this war on account of Spanish or any other kind of influenza."

In August of 1918, however, the influenza pandemic changed, as did the course of history. On a boat traveling from England to Sierra Leone in West Africa, nearly 200 of the crew were noted to be sick or recovering from the flu. After landing, the sick were taken to a local hospital. Within a week, the local dockworkers and other town members were sick, and, on one day alone, almost 85 percent of the coal loaders at the port were too ill to show for work and several died of pneumonia. Other ships arriving at Sierra Leone had similar concerns with large numbers of sick crew members; increasing numbers of deaths were reported.

Brest, another highly populated port in France, also began to suffer with a "new" version of influenza in mid- to late August of 1918. Ships with both American and French troops landed, allowing transmission of influenza from the sea crew to the population at the docks. In addition to the troops already afflicted with the flu, in the next three weeks, more than 1,300 natives were admitted to hospitals with influenza, and almost 400 died. Camps were created to deal with the increasing numbers of sick American army troops abroad (see Figures 3.1 and 3.2), but they were primitive and offered little containment of the disease. Spread of the illness throughout the rest of Europe followed quickly thereafter.

Back in the United States, several soldiers at Boston's Receiving Ship at Commonwealth Pier came down with flu symptoms and reported to their medical officers on August 27, 1918. Over the next forty-eight hours, the number of cases of influenza swelled to nearly seventy. Within a week, the number of affected would surpass 400, and, by the second week, nearly 2,000 were ill. Complicating the outbreak was the fact that life in the patriotic United States continued unchecked: war rallies and parades were ongoing, large numbers of young men were herded into indoor facilities to register for the draft, fans were

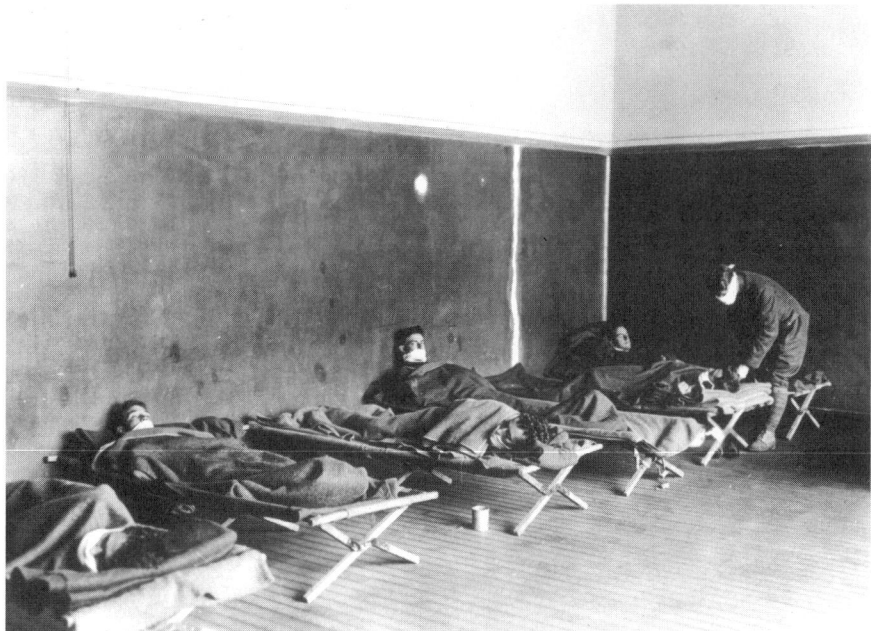

Figure 3.1. U.S. Army Field Hospital, No. 29. Interior view of the Influenza Ward of the U.S. Army Field Hospital, No. 29, in Hollerich, Luxembourg. Image used with permission from the 1918 Influenza Epidemic Gallery, courtesy of the National Museum of Health and Medicine, Armed Forces Institute of Pathology.

crowded into stadiums to watch sporting events (including the World Series, eventually won by the Boston Red Sox), and huge war bond parties were held. All of these events were perfect conditions for the spread of a highly infective virus like the latest influenza strain. By late September, the infection had spread across the United States, and outbreaks were reported at navy bases throughout the country. By the end of the month, more than 31,000 men ashore in the U.S. Naval Forces were sick with influenza, and at least 1,100 were dead.

On September 20, 1918, an article in the *New York Times* reported that Franklin D. Roosevelt (1882–1945) was afflicted with influenza:

> Franklin D. Roosevelt, Assistant Secretary of the Navy, who has been abroad for two months, arrived in New York yesterday and was taken to the home of his mother, Mrs. James Roosevelt, 47 East Sixty-fifth Street, suffering from a slight attack of pneumonia caused by Spanish influenza which he contracted on the ship, Mrs. Roosevelt said last night.

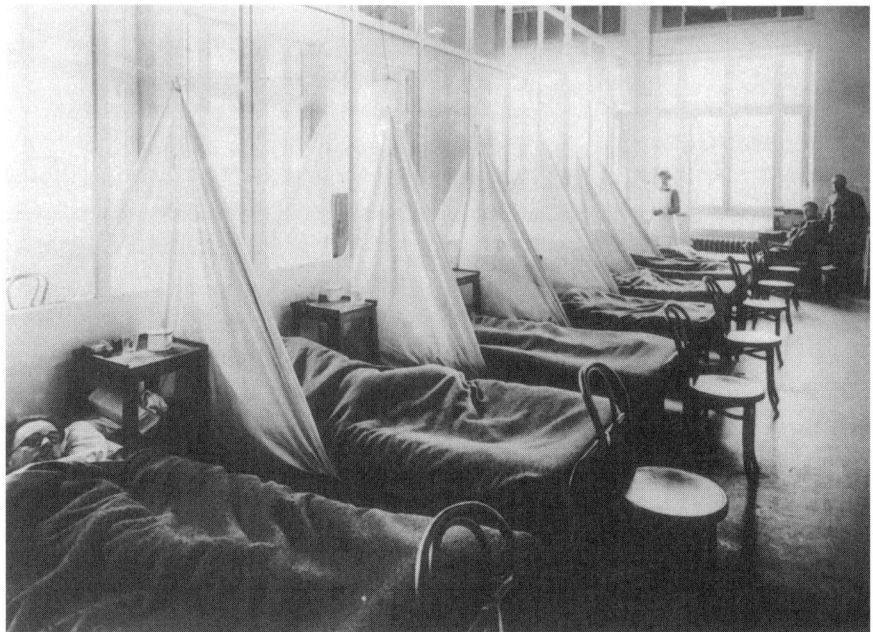

Figure 3.2. U.S. Army Camp Hospital, No. 45. Interior view of the Influenza Ward, No. 1, of the U.S. Army Camp Hospital, No. 45, Aix-Les-Bains, France. Image used with permission from the 1918 Influenza Epidemic Gallery, courtesy of the National Museum of Health and Medicine, Armed Forces Institute of Pathology.

It began to be apparent that this outbreak of influenza was different from the earlier attack in the spring of 1918. This second wave was severe, and, in addition to targeting the young and old (as influenza had been known to do in the past), it was attacking young healthy adults at a rate that had never before been observed. Furthermore, the young healthy adults were dying: a tenfold increase in the death rate among affected cases was documented. Even if death did not occur, the illness attributable to this wave of influenza infection was devastating, and the symptoms were horrific. Starting with the typical manifestations of fever, headache, cough, and malaise, patients progressed to a multitude of other symptoms, including (1) delirium with mental depression, hysteria, melancholy, or suicidal intent; (2) involuntary shaking; (3) neurological deficiencies; (4) agonizing muscle and joint pains; (5) profuse nausea and vomiting; (6) subcutaneous emphysema (pockets of air that accumulate just beneath the skin, which can be heard to "crackle" when pressure is applied); (7) extreme ear pain with perforation of the ear drum; (8) progressive pneumonia with respiratory failure and cyanosis (lack of oxygen to vital parts of the body, causing the skin to turn blue); (9) hemorrhaging of blood from the nose, mouth, ears, eyes, lungs, bowel, and even vagina; and (10) loss of eye movement and ability to smell.

Influenza Pandemic of 1918: Spotlight on Philadelphia

- In July, the Philadelphia Bureau of Health issued a bulletin, warning of the possible spread of influenza to the United States. Influenza reached the Naval Yard in mid-September, and, on September 18th, the Bureau of Health issued another warning about the disease. A public campaign against coughing, sneezing, and spitting was initiated. On September 21st, influenza was made a reportable disease.

- Despite influenza concerns, the Fourth Liberty Loan Drive was held on September 28th. Two hundred thousand people gathered together to watch a parade, sing songs, and buy bonds. After this event, the pandemic in Philadelphia exploded.

- On October 1st, 635 new cases of influenza (in civilians) were reported in a single day. By the end of the same week, 700 people were dead. In the next two weeks, another 7,100 were dead.

- City officials closed all places of amusement, including saloons and theaters, as well as schools and churches. The city was divided into seven districts to allow equal use of resources and classification of healthcare workers. All types of organizations and individuals rose to the challenge of fighting the disease, and amazing numbers of volunteers were assigned tasks to aid in handling both the sick and the dead.

- As quickly as it came, the influenza pandemic in Philadelphia began to wane. On October 27th, health authorities in Philadelphia lifted the ban on church services, and, the next day, schools were opened. By October 30th, theaters, saloons, and other businesses were opened as well.

- The American Red Cross reported that 54,038 flu masks, 20,444 bed sheets, 8,919 towels, and 605 pairs of pajamas were supplied to the people of Philadelphia during the pandemic. The closing of hotels, theaters, and saloons during the pandemic cost those businesses in excess of $2 million.

- Final mortality statistics, which surely underestimated the actual numbers because of inaccurate reporting during the crisis, revealed that 12,162 people in Philadelphia died between September 29th and November 2nd. Three peaks in the mortality curve were noted: those under five years of age, those between twenty-five and thirty-four years of age, and those over sixty-five years of age.

Katherine Anne Porter (1890–1980), previously a reporter for the *Rocky Mountain News*, was living in Denver when influenza swept through her city in 1918. She fell severely ill with the flu, and her fiancé, a young army lieutenant, cared for her until she was taken to a hospital. In her short novel, *Pale Horse, Pale Rider*, Porter's lead character, Miranda, becomes ill with influenza and hovers near death in a hallucinatory fever:

What is this whiteness and silence but the absence of pain? Miranda lay lifting the nap of her white blanket softly between eased fingers, watching a dance of tall deliberate shadows moving behind a wide screen of sheets spread upon a frame. It was there, near her, on her side of the wall where she could see it clearly and enjoy it, and it was so beautiful she had no curiosity as to its meaning. Two dark figures nodded, bent, curtsied to each other, retreated and bowed again, lifted long arms and spread great hands against the white shadow of the screen; then with a single round movement, the sheets were folded back, disclosing two speechless men in white, standing, and another speechless man in white, lying on the bare springs of a white iron bed. The man on the springs was swathed smoothly from head to foot in white, with folded bands across the face, and a large stiff bow like merry rabbit ears dangled at the crown of his head.

The two living men lifted a mattress standing hunched against the wall, spread it tenderly and exactly over the dead man. Wordless and white they vanished down the corridor, pushing the wheeled bed before them. It had been an entrancing and leisurely spectacle, but now it was over. A pallid white fog rose in their wake insinuatingly and floated before Miranda's eyes, a fog in which was concealed all terror and all weariness, all the wrung faces and twisted backs and broken feet of abused, outraged living things, all the shapes of their confused pain and their estranged hearts; the fog might part at any moment and loose the horde of human torments. She put up her hands and said, not yet, not yet, but it was too late. The fog parted and two executioners, white clad, moved towards her pushing between them with marvelously deft and practiced hands the misshapen figure of an old man in filthy rags whose scanty beard waggled under his opened mouth as he bowed his back and braced his feet to resist and delay the fate they had prepared for him. In a high weeping voice he was trying to explain to them that the crime of which he was accused did not merit the punishment he was about to receive; and except for this whining cry there was silence as they advanced. The soiled cracked bowls of the old man's hands were held before him beseechingly as a beggar's as he said, "before God I am not guilty," but they held his arms and drew him onward, passed, and were gone.

The road to death is a long march beset with all evils, and the heart fails little by little at each new terror, the bones rebel at each step, the mind sets up its own bitter resistance and to what end? The barriers sink one by one, and no covering of the eyes shuts out the landscape of disaster, nor the sight of crimes committed there. (Porter, 1939, 247–49)

Eventually, on her slow return to health, Miranda is able to open her waiting mail and reads then that her lover has died of influenza in a military hospital. This story has even more resonance when the reader realizes that it is autobiographical, and that Porter's soldier fiancé fell ill and died of influenza while she struggled against the infection. Porter herself was so near death that her newspaper had already set the type for her obituary. Luckily, although obviously with considerable consequences, she lived to write about it. As she would later say of the pandemic, "It just simply divided my life, cut across it like that." Porter took the title of her work from the words of an old song, "Pale horse, pale rider, done take my lover away," which may have had its influence from Revelations 6:8, in which Death, a pale rider on a pale horse, is given power "to kill with sword, and with hunger and with death, and with the beasts of the earth."

In January 1919, the pandemic reached Australia. It also spread throughout Africa and on to India. The pandemic was now truly global in its reach. India would become one of the areas hardest hit by the pandemic: it is estimated that 20 million may have perished on this subcontinent alone. In Cape Town, 4 percent of the population was dead of influenza in the first four weeks of infection. Ten percent of the population died in Chiapas, Mexico. In Brazil, attack rates reached 33 percent; in Buenos Aires, Argentina, attack rates exceeded 50 percent. In Japan, influenza sickened more than one third of the population. Both Russian and Iran would lose 7 percent of their entire population to influenza infection.

By the spring of 1919, the pandemic was barely perceptible. However, in January and February of 1920, the flu again made waves, but infection rates were less than in the previous two years. In the last week of January, more than 1,000 deaths were recorded in New York City and attributed to influenza and pneumonia. In February in Paris, 2,676 people died of influenza and/or pneumonia.

Vaccines were produced during the 1918 pandemic but were used with little success. Timothy Leary, a physician affiliated with Tufts Medical College, created the first influenza vaccine. It was distributed in small quantities to health departments of some of the United States' biggest cities and was then produced in larger amounts to allow mass vaccinations. Paul Lewis, the physician-scientist who was a mentor for Richard Shope at the Rockefeller Institute, was assigned the task of creating a vaccine for the 1918 influenza strain. Some of the vaccines seemed to hold promise and were produced in vast quantities. In San Francisco alone, 18,000 people were vaccinated before November 2, 1918. In the end, however, none of the vaccines offered much benefit beyond a placebo effect.

Influenza Pandemic of 1918: Spotlight on San Francisco

- Reacting to reports on the influenza pandemic arriving from the East coast, on September 21st, the Board of Health suggested that precautions against influenza be taken and that the area naval installations impose a quarantine.

- The first case of influenza in San Francisco was reported on September 24th in a gentleman who had traveled from Chicago. The next day, the second case was reported at a naval yard.

- On September 27th, influenza was made a reportable disease. The next day, San Francisco held its Fourth Liberty Loan Drive, and, over the next two weeks, hundreds of thousands of citizens attended rallies, marches, and speeches.

- On October 14th, 991 cases of flu were reported; by the end of the week, 4,000 new cases were identified. All places of amusement and public gathering were closed on October 18th; two days later, churches were closed as well.

- The city was divided into twenty districts to best use the available healthcare workers, hospital beds, and ambulances. These districts were redivided three more times until twelve districts remained. All districts were short of doctors, nurses, telephones, supplies, and volunteers.

- The number of active cases of influenza peaked on October 25th. In the two months after the start of the pandemic in San Francisco, 23,558 cases of flu were reported (likely an underestimate of actual cases). In October alone, 1,067 deaths were reported. Between October of 1918 and January of 1919, more than 50,000 cases of influenza were reported, with deaths exceeding 3,500. Two thirds of those who died were between the ages of twenty and forty years.

- On November 25th, the outbreak was considered ended when all public schools were reopened.

Besides vaccinations, other treatment modalities were attempted. Medical journals published claims from physicians of successful treatments for influenza: one required blowing a mixture of irritating chemicals into the upper respiratory tract to stimulate the flow of mucus, whereas another "cure" involved ingestion of potassium citrate and sodium bicarbonate to turn the human body alkaline. Hydrogen peroxide was given intravenously. Patients were injected with typhoid vaccines in hopes that the immune system would be boosted. Quinine, a treatment for malaria, was given, although there was no evidence it had any effect on influenza. In other parts of the world, alternative treatments were tried. In Greece, mustard plasters were used to create blisters, which were then drained; the fluid was mixed with morphine, strychnine, and caffeine and then reinjected into the patient. In Italy, a doctor gave intravenous injections of mercuric chloride. Other physicians tried rubbing disinfectants under the arms and giving enemas of warm milk and creosote. In France, physicians returned to the processes of cupping (using a flame to absorb oxygen and create a vacuum in a glass container, then placing the container on a part of the body) and bleeding.

Attention to preventative measures was eventually given. Surgical masks, made of gauze, were worn over the nose and mouth and tied with strings at the back of the head. Eventually, laws were passed to make wearing of masks mandatory in many places. Preventative throat sprays were administered (see Figure 3.3). To discourage spread of the infection, even at a time of peak patriotism in support of the United States' effort in the war, cancellation of rallies, bond parties, draft signings, parades, and military services was mandated. Businesses and schools were closed, and movie houses and theaters were shut down.

Influenza touched even the lives of celebrities at the time, as in the case of Harold Lockwood (1887–1918). He was born in Newark, New Jersey, and although his father wanted him to enter into a sales profession, Lockwood's heart remained true to the theater. As an adolescent, he performed as an extra on stage when his family moved to Manhattan. Eventually, he worked his way into musical comedy and vaudeville. Lockwood furthered his career as he became known to influential directors of the time, and, ultimately, he was paired onscreen with May Allison. The handsome, congenial Lockwood and the beautiful, talented Allison had amazing chemistry, and they starred in more than twenty consecutive films together between the years of 1915 and 1917. In June of 1918, Lockwood became the author of a popular monthly column entitled *Funny Happenings in the Studio and on Lockwood*. In early October of 1918, Lockwood became ill with influenza. By October 19, he was dead, at only thirty-one years of age. Other famous lives cut short by influenza in 1918 include Admiral Dot, a dwarf who was a member of P.T. Barnum's Great

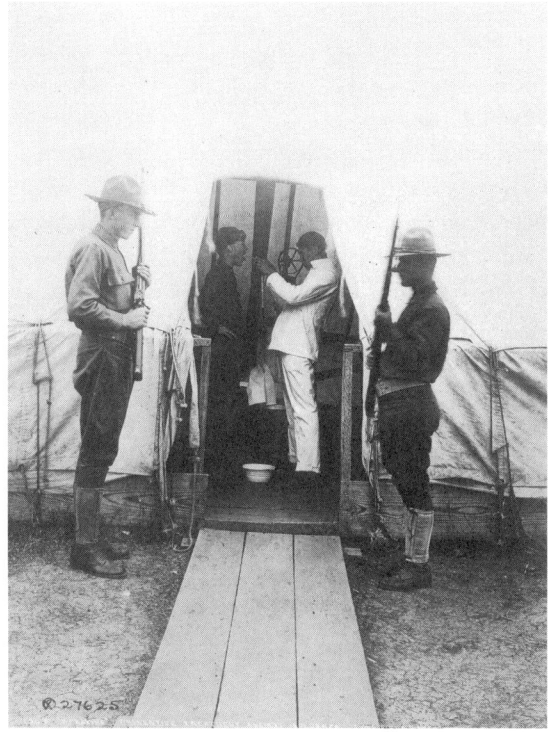

Figure 3.3. Preventative Treatment against Influenza. American Red Cross worker spraying the throat of a soldier in an attempt at preventative treatment of influenza at Love Field, Texas, November 6, 1918. Image used with permission from the 1918 Influenza Epidemic Gallery, courtesy of the National Museum of Health and Medicine, Armed Forces Institute of Pathology.

Traveling World's Fair, and Irma Cody Garlow, the youngest daughter of Buffalo Bill Cody (Irma's husband Fred also succumbed to the illness).

Ultimately, the total death toll attributed to the entire pandemic was astronomical. In the United States, over one-quarter of the population suffered from the flu during 1918–1919. Certain populations, such as the U.S. Navy, suffered in greater numbers; 40 percent of naval personnel had influenza in 1918, and more than 43,000 American sailors and soldiers died of the flu and pneumonia in that same year. In all of North America, 600,000 people died, including 25 percent of the population in Samoa and Alaska. Twenty-four percent of American Indians suffered from the flu between October 1918 and April 1919; 9 percent died. Pregnant women had death rates estimated to be up to 71 percent, and, of those pregnant women who survived, 26 percent lost their babies. Immigrants had a higher death rate from the flu and pneumonia than people born in the United States. In England and Wales, the official death count numbered 200,000. Worldwide, the estimated death toll was thought to potentially be 100 million.

GLOBAL INFLUENCE OF THE PANDEMIC

In addition to the astounding number of deaths and the effect on the world's population (particularly its young, healthy adults), the influenza pandemic of 1918 influenced many aspects of life in the early decades of the 1900s. At the peak of the deadly second wave of infection, the number of ill and dying patients far outweighed the available medical personnel needed to care for them. Because of severe shortages, physicians and nurses, regardless of background or training, were recruited to help deal with patients. In San Jose, California, one physician named W. Fowler apparently saw 525 patients in a single day during the peak epidemic. A recent reprint of an essay, first published in the *Annals of Internal Medicine* in 1976 by Isaac Starr, M.D., reveals an American medical perspective of life during the 1918 pandemic:

The summer of 1918 fell between the second and third years of my course at the University of Pennsylvania School of Medicine. Medical school opened as usual in mid-September. At the first of the regular Friday medical conferences the Professor of Medicine, Dr. Stengel, abandoned the usual schedule to lecture on influenza. From experience with the previous epidemic of 1888, he described the three main forms of the disease, those in which pulmonary, gastrointestinal, or nervous symptoms predominated. His suggestions for treatment were negative; he believed that the use of coal-tar derivatives such as phenacetin and acetanilide was contraindicated; he had no confidence in any of the remedies that had been proposed. On the following Monday morning the dean announced than an epidemic was judged to be developing and that, with so many medical practitioners away in the army, our services were needed in caring for the sick. So, for the third and fourth year classes, the medical school closed. I soon found myself "head nurse" on the top floor for the shift starting at 4 P.M. and ending at midnight.

Soon the beds were full, but nobody on my floor was very ill. The patients had fever but little else. Unhappily the clinical features of many soon changed drastically. As their lungs filled with rales the patients became short of breath and increasingly cyanotic. After gasping for several hours they became delirious and incontinent, and many died struggling to clear their airways of a blood-tinged froth that sometimes gushed from their nose and mouth. It was a dreadful business.

Thus my patient who often entered the ward with what appeared to be a minor illness became in a few days delirious and incontinent, gasping for breath and deeply cyanotic. After a day or two of intense struggle, they died. The deaths in the hospital as a whole exceeded 25% per night during the peak of the epidemic.

While this was going on in my ward, the life of the city had almost stopped. Public assembly was forbidden, so there were no plays, movies, concerts, or church services. Schools were closed. Some stores and businesses stayed open, some did not. All train schedules were reduced to those of Sunday, and these could not always be kept.

After about two weeks the deaths on the top floor began to diminish, and then they diminished rapidly. A mild febrile disease, identified as part of the epidemic only by the fact that there was no other explanation for it, appeared in the population with decreasing frequency for the next few weeks. I came down with this myself and was sick for a few days only. So, as mysteriously as it had come, the killer departed. At the height of the epidemic about one fifth of the total population of the emergency hospital died *each night*. (Starr, 2006, 138–140)

Beyond the healthcare establishment issues in the United States, other services were tested to capacity as more Americans fell ill. A lack of healthy telephone workers prompted newspaper ads to be placed by the Bell Telephone Company, warning customers that "no other than absolutely necessary calls compelled by the epidemic or by war necessity" would be handled. Fireman and policemen were too ill to show for work. Garbage collectors were unable to perform their duties, and trash piled in the sidewalks and streets. Children who watched their parents become sick with influenza and eventually die were left as orphans, and neighbors were asked to take them in. A catchy rhyme popular with children circulated quickly:

I had a little bird,
Its name was Enza.
I opened the window,
And in-flew-enza.

The morticians, undertakers, coffin manufacturers, and gravediggers were either too sick or too overwhelmed by the body counts, and the dead were left in their homes for days before a funeral or burial could take place. Morgues were filled to capacity, and bodies were piled on top of one another in rooms and hallways.

Colonel Charles Hagadorn, commander of Camp Grant in Rockford, Illinois, had devoted his life to the army. In an attempt to combat the overflowing population of soldiers at the camp in 1918, Hagadorn ignored warnings about overcrowding and issued orders to authorize filling of the barracks beyond recommended capacities. Within one day of issuing his orders, influenza struck the camp. On the day of the first reported soldier death, Hagadorn authorized a train of 3,108 troops to leave for Camp Hancock, just as a civilian health official demanded quarantine of his entire camp. Thousands at Camp Grant became infected with influenza, and the death toll exceeded 500. At least 10 percent of the troops on the train died of influenza, and the disease traveled to Camp Hancock undiminished. Hagadorn himself became a casualty of the epidemic by taking his own life in early October of 1918.

One global community touched by influenza was that of the art world, and influences from the time still exist today. In 1918, Egon Schiele (1890–1918) was a young but successful artist. According to his contemporaries, Schiele was the predestined successor to Gustav Klimt, but influenza unfortunately changed his fate. Schiele was born in Austria, and his early teen years were marked by the death of his father and a dislike of his mother. His attention as a late adolescent was thus focused on his younger sister Gerti. At age sixteen, Schiele was admitted to the Academy of Fine Arts in Vienna. The following year, he met his mentor, Klimt, who provided support by buying or trading Schiele's drawings, arranging models, and introducing him to potential patrons. After his third year at the academy, Schiele left to set up his own studio. His subjects of interest ran toward younger females, and he also made large numbers of self-portraits. In April of 1912, Schiele was arrested, and more than one hundred "pornographic" drawings were taken into custody. Ultimately, he was found guilty only of "exhibiting an erotic drawing in a place accessible to children." He served twenty-four total days in custody. During his imprisonment, Schiele produced an additional series of self-portraits (see Figure 3.4); one of these portraits was inscribed with the words, "To restrict the artist is a crime. It is to murder germinating life."

In June of 1915, Schiele married a young girl named Edith and spent the next several years in the military. In 1918, he participated in the Sezession's 49th Exhibition, and the show was considered a great triumph. On October 19th of that year, Edith, known to be pregnant, fell ill with fever and respiratory complaints. By October 28th, she was dead from infection with the influenza virus. Although their marriage had not been perfect, Schiele was

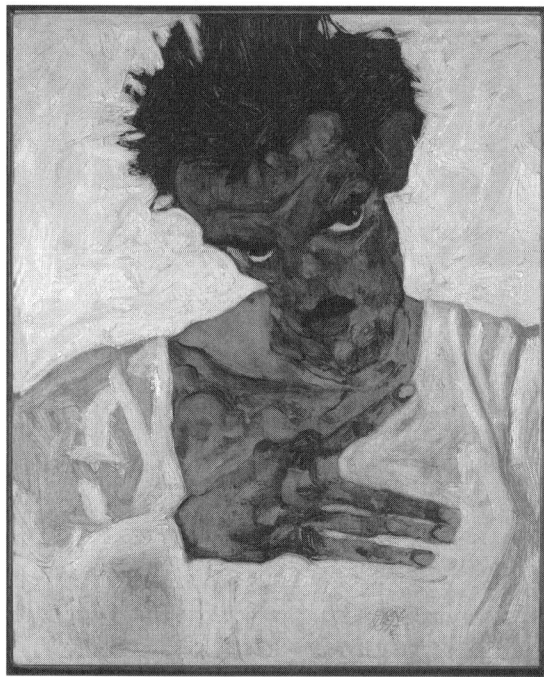

Figure 3.4. Self-Portrait with Bent Head, 1912. Egon Schiele's self-portrait, study for "Eremiten" (hermits), oil on wood, Museum Leopold, Vienna, Austria. Erich Lessing / Art Resource, NY.

devastated by her death. When he, too, fell ill with the flu, he managed to live only three days beyond his wife and passed away on October 31, 1918.

Another artist influenced by the 1918 influenza pandemic was Edvard Munch. Unlike Schiele, Munch managed to survive his bout with influenza, but it did affect him in ways that were best expressed by his paintings at the time. Munch has described himself as a sickly child, and he was influenced by death in childhood with the passing of both his mother and sister before he was fourteen. Munch was fifty-five years old when he fell ill with influenza. He was at the height of his fame and fortune when he painted *Self-Portrait after the Spanish Influenza* in 1919. M. Therese Southgate, M.D., in her cover editorial in the *Journal of the American Medical Association*, published in October of 2005, described it as follows:

> In a sense *Self-portrait After the Spanish Influenza* is Kierkegaard in Technicolor, in somber colors to be sure, and muted lest they make too much noise, but in color nonetheless; more remarkable, the work is deeply,

luxuriously sensual. In the foreground, filling most of the canvas, looms the hulking mass of a man in rich, variegated colors of blue, green, black, and brown. The figure is eerie, haunting, haggard, emaciated, still fever-demented perhaps, a Lazarus come out of the tomb, a ghost looking for its home. Under the too-large dressing gown, sagging shoulders describe near-perfect curves; heavy-lidded, almond-shaped eyes peer out of deep sockets, not trusting what the see; lips are thick, parched; the hair is shaggy, the beard untrimmed; the complexion as fiery as that of a devil's. The arms hang inertly at the sides, too heavy to raise. The eyes focus on nothing, as though to do so would be too great an effort. A triangle of brilliant though partially shadowed white emphasizes the gloom of the figure but also suggests a return to health. The remainder of the canvas points also to a more normal world: the familiar room with its multicolored carpet, the warm, brown furniture, the books, the pale green wall, the lines emphasizing not curves that lead nowhere except back to themselves, but straight and true diagonals and verticals that have the potential to stretch on forever. The carpet is notable for its contrasting through muted reds and greens, both colors significant to Munch. One of his persistent memories of childhood was the lights and colors of the Christmas of his fifth year. Shortly afterward, his mother died. Later, Munch would note that in his lexicon of color, red always denoted blood, life, passion, while green was the color of death. Finally, at the upper left a white rectangular patch indicates light entering from outside. In what would become a familiar shorthand of Munch, the window panes are indicated by a rudimentary tau cross. "Sickness is hell," says Munch. But to capture it on canvas is to triumph. (Southgate, 2005, 1733)

The art world, despite such devastation during the 1918 pandemic, would also relish an amazing collection of works that was dedicated to the memory of an influenza victim. James and Duncan Phillips were brothers of the closest kind. During their formative years, both brothers developed a love of contemporary art and art collecting. By 1916, James had been granted a yearly stipend from the family to add regularly to their collection. In the fall of 1918, James became ill, and, on October 21st, he died at the family home in Washington, D.C., of complications from influenza infection. Devastated by the loss of his brother, Duncan wrote the following:

There came a time when sorrow all but overwhelmed me. Then I turned to my love of painting for the will to live. Art offers two great gifts of emotion—the emotion of recognition and the emotion of escape. Both emotions take us out to the boundaries of self ... So in 1918 I incorporated the Phillips Memorial Gallery ... to create a memorial worthy of ... my father ... and my brother James Laughlin Phillips, an idealist ... a keen student of men and social conditions—a broad-minded, warm-hearted, lovable, and very noble American.

The Phillips Collection, still in existence, now has an inventory of nearly 2,500 pieces and includes works by famous artists, including Van Gogh, Matisse, O'Keefe, and others. It is housed in the Phillips family residence in Washington, D.C., the very site where James passed away (Morens and Taubenberger, 2006, 78–80).

There is no doubt that the political picture of 1918–1920 was also shaped by the influenza pandemic, particularly as the world attempted to move toward a resolution of World War I. On November 11, 1918, a peace armistice was signed and the war was officially declared over. Fifteen million had lost their lives in battle, and the war had caused great devastation and damage worldwide. Near the end of that year, President Woodrow Wilson joined his Chief Aid Edward House in France to participate in the Paris Peace Conference, meant to establish new relationships for the world's great powers. While there, House developed influenza and was sick in his room for ten days. Although he rallied his strength, his recovery was slow. Unfortunately, House had a relapse in illness. His participation in the peace conference was certainly affected, and his influence on President Wilson during the negotiations was likely compromised by his illness. In addition to House, several other members of the American envoy in France fell ill: Charles Seymour (protégé of House and future president of Yale University), James T. Shotwell (Columbia University historian and American aide), Norman Davis (American financier and diplomat), and Donald P. Frary (American Peace Commission's assistant librarian) all became ill with flu or pneumonia. On one day of illness during the conference, the American delegation doctors made 125 sick calls.

In April of 1919, President Woodrow Wilson abruptly became ill with fever, hoarseness, cough, shortness of breath, weakness, and diarrhea. The president's physician diagnosed influenza. Although he survived, Wilson was bedridden for almost five days. His associates also noted that his cognitive abilities seemed affected by the illness. Negotiations among the world leaders continued in his absence with the still-weakened House as his representative. Ultimately, Wilson strayed far from his preconference principles and goals, and it is quite likely that influenza and illness affected the Americans' ability to negotiate effectively in the signing of the Treaty of Versailles.

FACTORS INFLUENCING SEVERITY OF DISEASE

In the midst of the 1918 pandemic, many patriots in America postulated that the virus must have been a weapon of some kind, unleashed by the German enemy in World War I, leading some to suggest that the illness be named "the German Plague." Others theorized that war itself must have led to the appearance of the pandemic as a result of poisoned air from use of gas or as an effect of the putrifying dead. Of course, it is now quite clear that a naturally occurring influenza virus was responsible for the pandemic. Analysis of the 1918 viral genome suggests that the strain was derived wholly from an ancestor that originally infected birds and then adapted to humans. There is still ongoing research to understand why the virus was so deadly. Some of the factors that might have influenced the severity of the pandemic are listed below, although not all are able to explain completely why the virus so readily attacked and killed healthy, young adults.

Exaggerated Host Response

It is now thought that the vigorous proinflammatory immune response triggered by infection of young, healthy adults may have played a role in their unexpected and untimely deaths during the 1918 pandemic. Influenza viruses made today via recombinant techniques containing the HA and NA glycoproteins from the 1918 strain demonstrate a profound host response, followed by severe lung pathology and inflammation, in mice; the findings appear to be related to enhanced levels of alveolar macrophages, cytokines, and neutrophils. This host response may have led to ARDS in victims of the 1918 pandemic. Without the aid of intensive care medical treatment at the time, this disease process would routinely have been fatal.

Female Gender

Women suffered disproportionally during the pandemic of 1918, most prominently in India. This has been suggested to be a result of the physical strain of pregnancy or the demands of acting as caretakers for others. Additional concerns with regard to the clinical manifestations and severity of disease during influenza infection while pregnant will be discussed in Chapter 4.

Lack of Immunity

Sir MacFarlane Burnet (1899–1985), the 1960 recipient of the Nobel Prize for Medicine, postulated that the 1918 flu virus was a very virulent strain to which few humans had ever been exposed. If so, there would have been little resistance to infection with the virus among the general population. He felt that those born before 1889 or 1890 may have enjoyed some immunity as a result of previous exposure to influenza outbreaks, thus allowing the 1918 strain to preferentially infect and kill younger aged victims. Burnet also put blame on host factors: he felt that a young adult immune system might respond vigorously to sudden trauma, and that the response may lead to inflammation of the lungs when involved with the influenza virus.

Poor Leadership

Complacency, incompetency, or sickness may have left many federal, state, and city leaders unable to react to the pandemic in a timely manner. This could have ultimately influenced the death rates.

Secondary Bacterial Infection

There is a fairly high likelihood that many of the deaths in 1918 resulted from the combined effect of the influenza virus itself, followed by a subsequent bacterial pneumonia. Autopsy analysis and bacteriological examination of the lung tissue of influenza victims showed evidence of Pfeiffer's bacilli in many cases. Ernest W. Goodpasture (1886–1960), a pathologist at the Chelsea Naval Hospital near Boston, examined sixteen cadavers during the worst months of the 1918 pandemic. He found *Streptococcus pneumoniae* in the lungs of all but Pfeiffer's bacillus in only two. He postulated that a secondary streptococcal infection might have caused the death of some of the 1918 victims. Poor nutrition (possibly influenced by damage to crops from unusually severe monsoon rains during the same time period), lack of adequate housing, and a slimmer chance for supportive care may have allowed more bacterial super-infections to occur as well.

Richard Shope, the physician-scientist described in Chapter 1 for his work with swine flu, postulated that a synergistic cause was responsible for the pandemic of 1918. He theorized that the flu virus alone caused the first wave of influenza during the pandemic, but that the inclement weather of fall and the spread of Pfeiffer's bacillus may have triggered the virus into more virulent activity for the second deadly wave.

Shortages of Healthcare Providers

As described in the previous section, there were considerable shortages of healthcare providers in the United States, and the same inadequate numbers were documented across the globe as the pandemic reached its peak. The sick outnumbered the available help, leading to deficiencies in adequate fluids, food, and care, all of which may have increased the risk of death.

Underlying Disease

Influenza may also have influenced the underlying disease processes in some patients already suffering from diabetes, or heart and kidney problems, leading to an increased likelihood of organ failure and death.

In an attempt to study the influenza virus that resulted in the 1918 pandemic and to understand better the factors leading to its swift attack rate and astounding mortality, researchers have had to perform extraordinary feats. John Hultin, born in Stockholm, is one such scientist. His childhood, although privileged, was marked by tragedy. One of two sisters died at six months of age from an infection that entered the bloodstream after spreading from a wound on her finger, whereas the other sister died in a traumatic accident when she was only thirty-two. When Hultin was ten, his parents divorced, and he went to live with his mother and her second husband, Carl Naeslund. Naeslund was a professor of medicine at the Karolinska Institute in Stockholm, and he was a great influence on Hultin's growing passion for science and medicine. Hultin eventually traveled to Iowa for graduate study. It was here that Hultin's future became linked with the world of influenza.

Hultin proposed that he might be able to find influenza victims from the pandemic of 1918 who had been buried in permafrost in Alaska and, after excavating the bodies, extract the virus from their tissue for study. Hultin applied to the National Institutes of Health (NIH) for a research grant that would allow him to travel to Alaska, but was not notified for months. Eventually, he realized that the army had found his idea intriguing and was planning an expedition with the help of NIH. With that information in hand, Hultin was quickly granted an allowance by his university, and he left immediately for Alaska with a number of colleagues.

Hultin's search for the perfect permafrost conditions that were required for tissue salvage took him first to Nome and then to Wales. Although cemeteries and mass graves were identified with likely victims of the 1918 influenza pandemic, digs in those areas revealed a lack of permafrost. With no permafrost, the corpses were fully deteriorated, and no viable tissue or virus could be found. Hultin's last chance to find permafrost and, in turn, the influenza virus, was Brevig. Seventy-two of eighty people living in Brevig in 1918 had died of the flu in November of that year, and the bodies were buried in a mass grave. With the permission of the town's current inhabitants, Hultin began digging.

At three feet, he encountered permafrost. After four long days of work, Hultin found his first flu victim. According to Hultin, "she was a little girl, about six to ten years old." With the help of his excavation team, he eventually uncovered four other bodies.

They carefully removed small pieces of frozen lung tissue from each body and placed them in sterile containers. When this job was done, they closed the grave and returned to the University of Iowa. Once there, Hultin began to isolate the virus from the frozen lung tissue. He started by grinding up the tissue, suspending it in a salt solution, and spinning it in a centrifuge to separate the virus from debris. He then added an antibiotic to the fluid to try to kill any bacteria that may have been present, and from there began the tedious work of injecting the fluid into fertilized chicken eggs. After injecting hundreds of eggs, he watched for signs of viral growth. None ever came. Other suspensions obtained from the lung tissue were injected into the nasal passages of guinea pigs, white mice, and ferrets. Nothing happened. The animals remained healthy, and Hultin's supply of preserved tissue specimens was gone. The virus, unfortunately, was "dead." After all of his work, Hultin never wrote up his results or published a scientific paper on the failed experiment. As Hultin said, "If it had been positive it would be tremendous, but it was negative."

Another scientist intrigued by the subject of influenza was Jeffrey Taubenberger. Although Taubenberger was a relatively unknown researcher, he had access to the Armed Forces Institute of Pathology. During his tenure as president of the United States, Abraham Lincoln had mandated that every military doctor who examined tissue after a patient's death had to send a specimen to be stored in the repository at the Armed Forces Institute of Pathology. Taubenberger, born in Germany to a father who was a career army officer, settled in northern Virginia when his father was posted at the Pentagon. From a young age, he knew he wanted to be a scientist, and he skipped his senior year of high school to enroll at George Mason University in Fairfax. During the summers of his adolescent years, he got a job at the NIH, working on tumor viruses. After college, he entered the Medical College of Virginia in Richmond, studying medicine and microbiology simultaneously, and graduated with both an M.D. and a Ph.D. He then proceeded to a pathology residency at the National Cancer Institute, a part of the NIH. Taubenberger eventually became chief of the Division of Molecular Pathology.

With access to the available specimens in the repository, Taubenberger found seventy specimens from people who had died of the flu in 1918. Along with the specimens, he found medical records that described the clinical circumstances surrounding each patient's demise. Six of the victims were analyzed. On March 19, 1995, Taubenberger and his team began their work and managed to separate the genetic pieces of the 1918 virus from the tissue samples. They then moved to a technique called polymerase chain reaction (PCR), which allowed millions of copies to be made from a single fragment of a gene. The first experiment, and many more attempts, failed. Eventually, with help from an expert in isolation techniques, Taubenberger and his team managed to sequence a specimen from a victim of influenza in 1957. With a success in hand, they returned to a single victim from the 1918 flu: Roscoe Vaughan. Vaughan had been a twenty-one-year-old soldier at Camp Jackson in South Carolina in September of 1918. His medical record indicated he had a rapid onset of illness with high fever, chest pain, and cough. He had also died very suddenly, and his lungs on autopsy showed that his air sacs were filled with fluid. The records seemed to suggest that indeed flu had been the cause of his death, not a secondary process such as bacterial pneumonia. With Vaughan's specimens, Taubenberger and his team matched one viral gene after another for influenza: the NA, the MI, the M2, and finally the HA. Thus, the strain of influenza causing the 1918 pandemic was identified: H1N1. Taubenberger and his team published a paper in *Science*, announcing their findings to the world.

Scientists have now studied the 1918 viral strain extensively. When this virus was introduced into chicken embryos, it was lethal. When introduced into mice, it caused severe disease, and all of the animals were dead within five days. It also showed a high propensity and great ability for replication in the lung cells of humans. Some of the factors now thought to have contributed to the particular lethality of the 1918 strain are (1) higher replication and higher virulence of the HA gene; (2) enhanced pathogenicity of the virus and allowance of trypsin-independent activation of HA by the NA gene; (3) faster replication in human respiratory epithelial cells and in the lungs of mice attributable to polymerase proteins PB1, PB2, and PA; and (4) inhibition of the host's interferon response attributable to a nonstructural protein, encoded by the NS1 gene, that contributes to replication and pathogenicity. Amazingly, when compared with the more contemporary strains of H1N1 influenza, the 1918 virus produced 39,000 times more virus particles in the lungs of mice! Some of the amino acid changes identified in the 1918 strain have also been seen in the H5N1 and H7N7 avian influenza viruses that have more recently been implicated in human fatalities.

After learning of Taubenberger's work, John Hultin returned to Alaska in the late 1990s on a solo expedition to attempt recovery of additional tissue specimens from the 1918 pandemic. He returned to the same village at Brevig and began to dig. After four days, he encountered the corpse of a young woman, Lucy, who had perished of influenza in her twenties during the pandemic. Opening her chest, Hultin found that her lungs remained frozen, and that they were filled with blood. Carefully preserved specimens were taken and ultimately shipped in separate packages to the Armed Forces Institute of Pathology. In just ten days' time, Hultin was informed that genetic material from the 1918 virus had been isolated from his tissue specimens. His work was instrumental in allowing the sequencing of the 1918 influenza genome. Hultin later said,

> I knew it, I knew the virus was there. That was one of the great days for me. The virus sat and waited for me. Maybe it was good I didn't find it before, technology wasn't ready for it yet. Also, if I had found it, I would have become a famous person. My future would have been very narrow. I didn't find it, so I had the chance to do other things.

SIGNIFICANCE OF THE PANDEMIC FOR TODAY

As said by George Santayana in 1905, "Those who cannot remember the past are condemned to repeat it." An increase in the incidence of avian influenza worldwide in both poultry and humans raises the obvious concern of the likelihood of another influenza pandemic. Most medical experts agree that it is not a matter of if, but when. Since the 1918 pandemic, the world's population has grown threefold; if a new viral strain causing a pandemic is to be as lethal as the 1918 strain in today's age, it could kill as many as 180–360 million people. More conservative estimates place the potential death toll of a future pandemic at 62 million. In either case, such a pandemic would certainly overwhelm the existing healthcare systems worldwide and have a devastating socioeconomic impact from a global perspective.

Although medical advances have certainly been made since 1918, today's population is increasingly at risk for a great pandemic from a disease such as influenza. Some of the vulnerabilities include the following:

- An outbreak in a remote village can be spread to major cities of the world in days thanks to advances in transportation.
- More people are alive today with immune system compromise (elderly, infirm, those with compensated chronic diseases, and transplant patients), putting them at risk for greater rates of complications and mortality, as well as preferential spread of the infection to others.
- Public health infrastructures have not kept pace with growing vulnerabilities.

As outlined in the previous chapter, the most pressing recent concern is the avian influenza strain identified as H5N1. This virus has already jumped from aquatic birds to poultry to humans with impressive mortality rates and spread from human to human may be possible. Although the exact origin of the 1918 virus has not yet been made clear, most hypotheses suggest that it may have evolved from an avian virus that adapted to infect humans. Some of the amino acid changes in the 1918 strain that could be potential contributors to its human adaptation have also been identified during study of the H5N1 strain.

The H5N1 strain continues to mutate: in 2002, it underwent genotypic changes that resulted in increased pathogenicity in ducks and aquatic fowl, and, in 2003, it mutated further and infected a family from Hong Kong. Most of the isolated H5N1 strains in humans have acquired a few changes in the HA, NA, polymerase, and NS1 genes and have caused a deregulated host response in the infected victims. With H5N1 still in circulation, the worry is that it will mutate enough to become capable of sustained transmission among humans, causing a new influenza pandemic of unpredicted virulence. Besides the H5N1 strain, other avian influenza viruses have successfully been transmitted from birds to humans, although, fortunately, most have not shown the lethality associated with H5N1.

PREPARATION FOR A FUTURE INFLUENZA PANDEMIC

In the United States, work of the U.S. Department of Health and Human Services (HHS), through its National Institute of Allergy and Infectious Diseases, to prepare for a possible future avian influenza pandemic is ongoing. Areas in which research and development are focused include the following:

- development of pre-pandemic vaccines based on current lethal strains of H5N1
- collaboration with pharmaceutical industry leaders to increase the nation's vaccine production capacity in the event of a pandemic
- research in the development of new types of influenza vaccines that might allow for prevention of or protection from a pandemic strain of influenza
- studies in the effectiveness of available antiviral medications for treatment of pandemic avian influenza

The HHS has an impressive presence in planning for the pandemic at national, state, and local levels within the United States. In addition to their role as a federal government agency, they have made pandemic planning checklists and toolkits available to state and local governments, law enforcement agencies, correctional facilities, businesses (including U.S. businesses located overseas), long-term care and residential facilities, schools, the health-care industry, community organizations, and individuals and families.

From a global perspective, the United States has also entered into a partnership with countries and international organizations around the world to prepare for and respond to the challenge of avian pandemic influenza. President George W. Bush announced the International Partnership on Avian and Pandemic Influenza during the United Nations General Assembly in September of 2005, with the following goals: (1) elevate the avian influenza issue on national agendas, (2) coordinate efforts among donor and affected nations, (3) mobilize and leverage resources, (4) increase transparency in disease reporting and improve surveillance, and (5) build local capacity to identify, contain, and respond to an influenza pandemic.

As of May of 2007, the United States had pledged $434 million to support international efforts for pandemic preparation and planning, and the global community in total has promised more than $1.8 billion. The United States works with more than fifty countries in collaboration with the WHO, the Food and Agriculture Organization, the World Organization for Animal Health, and other international and in-country partners on pandemic preparedness. Some of the collaborative efforts thus far have included, but are not limited to, the following:

- deployment of scientists, veterinarians, public-health experts, physicians, and emergency response teams to affected and high-risk countries to assist in the development and implementation of emergency preparedness plans and procedures
- collaboration with Canada and Mexico to develop a comprehensive North American plan for pandemic preparedness
- work with international organizations such as the World Bank and the Asian Development Bank, and regional forums such as the Asia Pacific Economic Cooperation forum, to strengthen preparedness
- enhancement of radio, television, and Internet coverage of international avian influenza outbreaks, and responses in English and dozens of other languages for Asia, Africa, and Latin America
- support of efforts to expand animal and human disease surveillance systems worldwide and work with international partners to improve capacity for detection and laboratory diagnosis, as well as early-warning networks, in approximately forty countries
- participation with the Influenza Genome Sequencing Project, a collaborative effort to increase the genome knowledge base of influenza to help efforts to develop new influenza vaccines and drugs

- provision of funds to strengthen WHO's global outbreak alert and response network for surveillance and response worldwide and establishment of a fund to ship specimens promptly to reference laboratories for additional diagnosis and confirmation
- provision of training for thousands of policy and technical experts globally who will lead efforts to contain and mitigate the impact of animal outbreaks
- deployment of personal protective equipment kits to seventy-one countries for use by surveillance workers and outbreak response teams
- stockpiling of antiviral medications in Asia for potential use in a pandemic
- participation with WHO in investigations into human cases of H5N1

For specific publications and website addresses dealing with both the United States' and the global response to the threat of avian pandemic influenza, see the Bibliography.

4

The Clinical Manifestations of Influenza

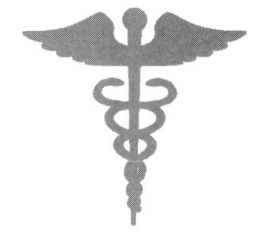

At eleven o'clock one of the Kansas men came to tell Claude that his Corporal was going fast. Big Tannhauser's fever had left him, but so had everything else. He lay in a stupor. His congested eyeballs were rolled back in his head and only the yellowish whites were visible. His mouth was open and his tongue hung out at one side. From the end of the corridor Claude had heard the frightful sounds that came from his throat, sounds like violent vomiting, or the choking rattle of a man in strangulation, and, indeed, he was being strangled. One of the band boys brought Claude a camp chair, and said kindly, "He doesn't suffer. It's mechanical now. He'd go easier if he hadn't so much vitality. The Doctor says he may have a few moments of consciousness just at the last, if you want to stay."

One of Ours, by Willa Cather, American Author, 1922

This passage, written by Willa Cather in her novel *One of Ours*, is a short but powerful description of the symptoms experienced by a dying soldier suffering from influenza during the influenza pandemic of 1918. Cather, a journalist-turned-novelist, became ill with influenza herself in the fall of 1919. A physician named Frederick Sweeney provided medical attention to Cather while she was sick. During their visits together, Dr. Sweeney told the author of his time aboard a troop ship bound for France during the second wave of the pandemic and admitted that he had kept a diary during those days. Eventually, Cather was given access to his diary, and she incorporated many of the details regarding the pandemic, its victims' sufferings, and the fatal outcomes into her fictional work.

Although such descriptions of the manifestations experienced during illness with influenza are impressive, it is not well understood by the afflicted that it is the consequences of the inflammatory cascade and the resulting host cell death that cause the actual symptoms rather than the circulation of the influenza virus through the system. The influenza virus, as has been mentioned previously, usually spreads from person to person in the aerosolized droplets that spew from the body during coughing, sneezing, or even talking. The droplets do not remain suspended in the air for long and travel less than one meter in most circumstances. Thus, transmission of the virus actually requires close contact between the source and the recipient, although it is possible that contact with surfaces contaminated with respiratory droplets might also allow infection. Once transported to a new host, the influenza virus binds to, and is taken in by, the ciliated epithelial cells along the respiratory tract. Viral replication ensues, and eventual necrosis and death of the host epithelial cell occurs. During this time, an inflammatory response in the host is triggered by recognition of the virion by the immune system, and production of antibodies and other protective substances begins, along with the identifiable clinical syndrome known as the flu.

After infection with the influenza virus has occurred, most patients will have an interval of time in which no symptoms are recognized; this is called the incubation period. Although the duration of the incubation period varies for each infectious agent, it typically lasts just a few days with influenza. In some lucky patients, little to no symptoms are ever appreciated, even beyond the incubation period. In most others, however, an abrupt onset of symptoms occurs once the incubation period is complete, signifying full activation of the immune defense system. Some cases of influenza remain uncomplicated, whereas others progress to more worrisome and severe manifestations or even death.

UNCOMPLICATED INFLUENZA

In uncomplicated cases of influenza, the symptoms are uncomfortable but rarely fatal. The most prominent manifestations of uncomplicated influenza might include the following: fever, chills or rigors, cephalgia, myalgias, fatigue or malaise, anorexia, tearing and/or burning of the eyes, arthralgias, and confusion and/or stupor.

These symptoms usually last about three days, although the fever can persist for four to eight days in some patients. The presence of fever is probably the

Clinical Manifestations of Uncomplicated Influenza

Fever: An elevation of the core body temperature above normal.

Chills or rigors: Involuntary shaking or tremors accompanied by a sense of coldness.

Cephalgia: An ache in the head.

Myalgias: An aching in the muscles, including extremities, the long muscles of the back, eye muscles (particularly when looking sideways), and calf muscles (primarily in children).

Fatigue and/or malaise: Overwhelming sense of exhaustion, often manifested by a difficulty getting out of bed.

Anorexia: Poor appetite with decreased ingestion of food and liquids.

Tearing and/or burning of the eyes: Watering from the eyes, or sense of heat or discomfort at the eyes.

Arthralgias: Pains in the joints.

Confusion and/or stupor: Changes in mentation or level of alertness, usually seen in elderly patients.

most important physical finding in identifying a patient with influenza. The temperature of an infected patient can rise suddenly and can reach as high as 106 degrees Fahrenheit within twelve hours. The fever is often continuous but occasionally may be intermittent (especially if medications to aid in fever reduction are used by patients; these medications are called antipyretics). In some patients, fever that appears to have resolved can recur again on the third or fourth day of symptoms, creating what is called a biphasic fever curve.

Although the previous description by Cather at the beginning of this chapter reveals a significant pulmonary component in the dying patient (indeed, observers of the sufferings experienced during the pandemic in 1918 often said that the dying patients appeared to be "drowning"), respiratory symptoms are usually present to a lesser extent than the systemic, or generalized, complaints in uncomplicated influenza. Respiratory complaints can include a dry cough (not associated with the production of sputum), throat pain, nasal congestion or discharge, and hoarseness or dry throat. In children, a "croupy" cough may be appreciated, with a sharp, barking quality to the cough. Often the respiratory symptoms persist three to four days beyond cessation of the fever. After this phase, a patient may take one to two, or more, weeks to entirely recover to his or her original state of baseline health. The last symptoms to fully resolve are often the cough and the sense of fatigue or malaise. Adults are infectious to others at least a day before onset of symptoms and can shed virus for up to five to seven days after symptom resolution.

The illness caused by influenza A is nearly indistinguishable from the illness caused by influenza B from the clinical perspective, although it has been suggested that influenza B might produce a somewhat milder illness than A. Influenza C, however, usually manifests only as a "cold" and rarely causes the host to suffer from the systemic symptoms described above.

COMPLICATED INFLUENZA

Although many cases of human influenza in recent years have been of the uncomplicated form, two types of pneumonia have been described in the setting of influenza infection that can lead to more serious consequences. Occasionally, a combination of the two types of pneumonia can exist in the same patient at the same time.

Primary Viral Pneumonia

The first type of pneumonia is attributable to the influenza virus itself and is called primary viral pneumonia. This illness often begins with the symptoms as already described for uncomplicated influenza. Unfortunately, the fever and cough can be quickly followed by a rapid progression to shortness of breath, increased work of breathing, and an inability to transport oxygen as needed to vital tissues. The lack of oxygen causes a bluish color to occur and can best be seen at the fingers and lips; this is known as cyanosis.

The risk of death in patients who progress to primary viral pneumonia is high. Unfortunately, antibiotics are not effective in treating this type of pneumonia because they do not have any killing activity against viruses. When autopsies are performed on influenza victims who have died of primary viral pneumonia, inflammation along the respiratory tract at the trachea, the bronchial tree, and into the alveolar ducts can be appreciated (see Figure 4.1). At the level of the air sacs of the lungs, few inflammatory cells are found. Evidence of bleeding along the respiratory tract can be seen, as well.

It is now suggested that many of the deaths occurring in patients during the 1918 and 1957 influenza outbreaks were attributable to this complication. In more recent epidemics, this syndrome has been seen in patients who suffer from underlying heart (specifically, stenosis of the mitral valve) or lung disease and in pregnant women.

Thomas Wolfe was a student at the University of North Carolina when his beloved brother Benjamin fell ill with influenza during the 1918 pandemic; Ben was quickly diagnosed with pneumonia. Wolfe returned home to see his brother

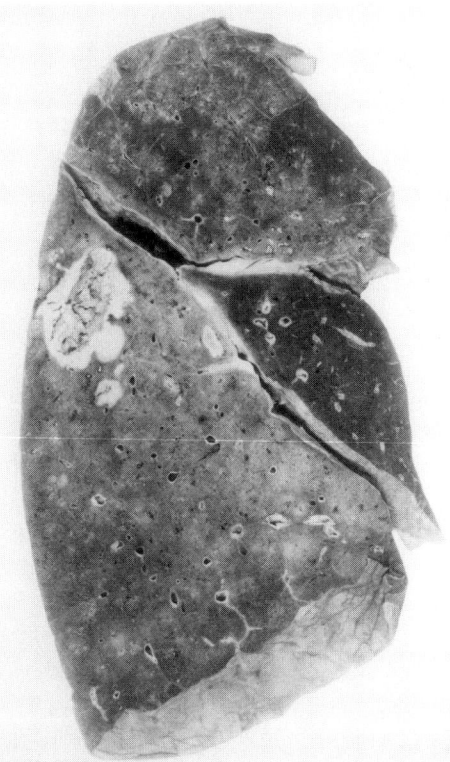

Figure 4.1. Pulmonary Autopsy Specimen, 1918. Autopsy specimen of the lung, dating to the influenza pandemic of 1918, depicting bronchopneumonia. Image used with permission from the 1918 Influenza Epidemic Gallery, courtesy of the National Museum of Health and Medicine, Armed Forces Institute of Pathology.

and, ultimately, was forced to watch helplessly as Ben succumbed to his illness. In his novel, *Look Homeward, Angel,* Wolfe revisits the experience:

> Ben's long thin body lay three-quarters covered by the bedding; its gaunt outline was bitterly twisted below the covers, in an attitude of struggle and torture. It seemed not to belong to him, it was somehow distorted and detached as if it belonged to a beheaded criminal. And the sallow yellow of his face had turned gray; out of this granite tint of death, lit by two red flags of fever, the stiff black furze of a three-day beard was growing. The beard was somehow horrible; it recalled the corrupt vitality of hair, which can grow from a rotting corpse. And Ben's thin lips were lifted, in a constant grimace of torture and strangulation, above his white somehow dead-looking teeth, as inch by inch he gasped a thread of air into his lungs.

And the sound of this gasping—loud, hoarse, rapid, unbelievable, filling the room, and orchestrating every moment in it—gave to the scene its final note of horror.

Ben lay upon the bed below them, drenched in light, like some enormous insect on a naturalist's table, fighting, while they looked at him, to save with his poor wasted body the life that no one could save for him. It was monstrous, brutal. (Wolfe, 1997, 460)

Secondary Bacterial Pneumonia

The second type of pneumonia described in influenza infection is that caused by bacteria rather than the influenza virus itself and is known as secondary bacterial pneumonia. While a host's immune system attempts to combat the viral infection, it can leave the unfortunate victim at risk for another infection caused by bacteria. The influenza virus inhibits adequate action of the disease-fighting white blood cells in the lungs themselves, so, if the host is exposed to bacteria, it may not be able to avoid new infection. There is also evidence that the influenza virus facilitates some bacteria's ability to attach to lung tissue and cause infection. Typical bacteria that might cause a secondary pneumonia now include *Staphylococcus aureus* or *Streptococcus pneumoniae*; however, *Haemophilus influenzae* (the updated name for Pfeiffer's bacillus) still exists and is known to complicate influenza infections to this day.

The patients who tend to suffer from secondary bacterial pneumonia are often at the extremes of age and may be ill with other diseases such as heart, lung, or metabolic problems. Usually, patients will have an identifiable illness attributable to influenza first and show a brief period of recovery over two to three days. Shortly thereafter, however, the victims will suffer again from symptoms, including fever, cough, production of purulent (resembling pus) sputum, and difficulty breathing. The patients may appear quite toxic and, if examined, can demonstrate signs of infection deep into the lungs during auscultation with a stethoscope. Their sputum, when evaluated in the laboratory, shows a predominance of bacteria, often with one in the majority as the primary pathogen. Because bacteria can be targeted with antibiotic therapy, these patients often get better with supportive care and appropriate antimicrobial medications. It has been proposed that, in addition to the prevalence of primary viral pneumonia, the severity of the second wave of the 1918 pandemic (and the tendency for the virus to kill young, healthy adults) was attributable to the possible synergy between the influenza virus itself and a complicating bacteria. This was the theory of Richard Shope; the bacteria he blamed as the causative agent was Pfeiffer's bacillus.

EXTRA-PULMONARY COMPLICATIONS OF INFLUENZA

Less frequently, complications outside of the respiratory tract have been described in patients infected with influenza. As was discussed in Chapter 3, the symptoms experienced by patients during the 1918 pandemic were often severe and all encompassing and could include the following: delirium with mental depression, hysteria, melancholy, or suicidal intent; neurological deficiencies; subcutaneous emphysema (pockets of air that accumulate just beneath the skin that can be heard to "crackle" when pressure is applied); extreme ear pain with perforation of the ear drum; hemorrhaging of blood from the nose, mouth, ears, eyes, lungs, bowel, and even vagina; and loss of eye movement and ability to smell.

Cardiac Complications

Inflammation of the heart muscle, known as myocarditis, and/or the heart lining, termed pericarditis, have been described in influenza infection. Although some patients have suffered from heart attacks while suffering from influenza, it is rare to see elevation of cardiac muscle enzymes or ischemic muscle damage during involvement of the heart in influenza.

Central Nervous Complications

Named after the French neurologists George Guillain (1876–1951) and Jean Alexander Barré (1880–1967), Guillain-Barré syndrome (GBS) has been described in patients who have suffered from influenza. GBS is an autoimmune disorder in which the host's immune system attacks its own nervous system. This causes varying degrees of muscle weakness and abnormalities in sensation that first start at the legs and, over time, may progress to the upper body and arms, eventually causing full paralysis and a need for total care and support. If the paralysis ascends to the level of the diaphragm and the nerves that influence respiration, patients may even require breathing assistance with a mechanical ventilator. GBS can develop within days to weeks after influenza infection, and it is not clear who is at risk for its occurrence; this makes any attempt at prevention of GBS difficult. Treatment for GBS is primarily supportive in nature, because the disorder will often improve over time and patients may recover completely. Unfortunately, however, some patients have residual neurological deficits once the acute illness has passed or may even die. Other treatments used now include plasmapheresis (removal of plasma from the sick patient and replacement with donor plasma) and infusion of high-dose immunoglobulins (antibodies).

Cases of transverse myelitis and encephalitis have also been reported in patients who have had influenza infection. Transverse myelitis refers to inflammation of the spinal cord along a cross-section, inducing neurological symptoms (often paralysis) below the level of involvement. Encephalitis is inflammation of the brain, often leading to confusion and/or stupor.

Conjunctivitis

Although red, teary eyes are not necessarily an uncommon finding in uncomplicated influenza, a more severe form of conjunctivitis can occur. Avian influenza H7N7 seems to have a predilection for conjunctival epithelium, and isolated conjunctivitis has been described in infections with this viral strain.

Croup

The term croup is used to describe a condition characterized by a barking cough, hoarseness, and stridor (a harsh sound heard during inspiration). It can occasionally be seen in children infected with influenza.

Myositis

Rarely associated with influenza B infection, and to a lesser extent with infection caused by influenza A, myositis refers to inflammation of the muscles. The median time to onset of myositis after identification of influenza infection is seventy-two hours. Most often, the calf muscles are involved, but other muscles groups are sometimes affected at the same time. The inflammatory process causes tenderness and an elevated muscle enzyme, known as creatine phosphokinase, detectable in a sick patient's blood when tested. Symptoms can be severe enough to prevent the patient from walking normally. Myositis has been most commonly reported in children, boys more often than girls; however, it can occur in adults as well. In most cases, the symptoms resolve in about three days, although a small number of patients may have persistence of symptoms for weeks.

Reye's Syndrome

This illness usually manifests as a combination of confusion and liver disease and can occur several days after a respiratory illness such as influenza. The most frequent laboratory abnormality seen in Reye's syndrome is elevation of ammonia in the blood. This syndrome has most often been connected with influenza B rather than influenza A. It has also been associated most strongly in children who were given aspirin to treat fever caused by influenza

Clinical Manifestations of H5N1 Avian Influenza

The clinical scenarios described in patients suffering from H5N1 avian influenza have ranged from a mild flu-like illness to a life-threatening disseminated disease process. Patients typically have fever, and respiratory symptoms can include congestion, cough, or difficulty breathing. Other reported symptoms include nausea, vomiting, diarrhea (a fairly prominent presenting symptom), headache, myalgias, sore throat, runny nose, conjunctivitis, and bleeding gums. Multi-organ failure with kidney dysfunction, compromise of cardiac function, pulmonary hemorrhage, collapse of the lung, and decreased blood counts are all complications that have been seen in infection with H5N1. The majority of deaths, however, have been attributed to respiratory failure.

- In the initial 1997 outbreak in Hong Kong, eight of the eighteen patients were children less than twelve years of age, and all but one had a relatively mild respiratory infection. The remaining patients had variable symptoms, including fever (100%), upper respiratory tract infection (67%), pneumonia (58%), and gastrointestinal symptoms (50%).
- In a report of ten Vietnamese and five Thai patients with H5N1, each initially suffered from fever and lower respiratory tract symptoms. All of the patients progressed to ARDS and died between six and twenty-nine days after presentation.
- In two children from Vietnam with identified H5N1 infection, diarrhea and confusion were the prominent symptoms. Both children died, and the virus was later identified in their cerebrospinal fluid, stool, throat, and blood.

or other viruses. The incidence of Reye's syndrome has decreased significantly now that patient education measures prevent the use of aspirin during acute respiratory illnesses in the pediatric population.

Toxic Shock Syndrome

It has been observed that some patients who acquire a secondary infection with *Staphylococcus aureus* bacteria while infected with influenza develop toxic shock syndrome (TSS). The influenza virus itself appears to change the replication characteristics of the toxin-producing bacteria. The toxins released into the system of the host can cause severe clinical consequences, including the following:

- high fever
- refractory drop in blood pressure
- redness of the eyes, lips, tongue, and throat

- rash resembling sunburn, even on the palms and soles
- nausea, vomiting, and/or diarrhea
- headache, confusion, and even seizure activity
- muscle aches

The treatment for TSS is hospitalization, antibiotics to target the *Staphylococcus aureus* bacteria, blood pressure support, and care for the other symptomatic complaints. Occasionally, the drop in blood pressure and toxin production of the bacteria can lead to kidney failure, and patients need to undergo a process known as dialysis. Rarely, the symptoms of TSS can be overwhelming, and death occurs.

Newer strains of influenza may allow a TSS-like syndrome to occur as a result of cytokine release. The exaggerated response of these cytokines can cause fever, chills, vomiting, and headache. More worrisome, however, is the ability of the cytokines to enhance the human immune response to the point of death.

INFLUENZA MANIFESTATIONS IN SPECIAL PATIENT POPULATIONS

At the extremes of age, differences in illness caused by influenza have been described. In addition, patients with underlying diseases or those undergoing treatments involving the immune system, lungs, heart, or kidneys may suffer more severely during an influenza infection.

Children

Younger patients are much more likely to become infected with influenza than adults. It has been estimated that 15–42 percent of preschool and school-aged children become infected with influenza each year, and these infections are associated with an increased number of outpatient healthcare visits, increased rates of hospitalization, more absences from school for both the patient and siblings, and many missed work days for parents. Temperatures can reach a higher level in children than adults. Swollen and tender lymph nodes at the neck are increasingly common in children as well. As was mentioned above, croup and Reye's syndrome can occur with influenza infection in children. Younger patients are also more likely to suffer from ear pain, nausea, and vomiting. Occasionally, they may actually have seizure activity occur when the fever is high; 6–20 percent of children hospitalized with influenza have been reported to have such febrile seizures.

Children are highly contagious with influenza: they may begin shedding the virus days before symptoms occur and continue to shed for more than ten days beyond the active phase of illness.

In very young children, or in children with certain medical conditions, influenza infection can be associated with an increased risk of hospitalization or severe complications. This includes children with the following disorders: (1) chronic pulmonary diseases, such as asthma, cystic fibrosis, or bronchopulmonary dysplasia (a lung disorder that can occur in premature infants); (2) conditions that compromise respiratory function or the ability to handle respiratory secretions, or increase the risk of aspiration, such as spinal cord injuries, seizure disorders, or neuromuscular conditions; (3) congenital heart disease; (4) hemoglobinopathies (disorders characterized by alterations in the structure of hemoglobin, which often results in anemia); (5) metabolic conditions, such as diabetes; and (6) conditions (such as cancer or human immunodeficiency virus [HIV] infection) or medications that cause immunosuppression. The incidence of both primary viral pneumonia and secondary bacterial lung infection requiring hospitalization is higher in these patients, and influenza shedding can be prolonged (up to weeks after symptoms resolve). When compared with older patients, children also experience a higher frequency of central nervous complications, which are often associated with very poor outcomes. Despite the increased risk of complicated disease in select pediatric patients, children are less likely to die of influenza infection than adults.

In an attempt to minimize the effects of influenza infection on children, the Advisory Committee on Immunization Practices (ACIP) of the CDC recommends routine influenza vaccination of children aged six to twenty-three months and has recently extended the recommendation to children up to five years of age. Older children have not previously been recommended for annual vaccination against influenza unless plagued by a chronic medical condition that puts them at increased risk for complications.

Chronic Disease Patients

People who suffer from chronic lung disease or asthma can have worsening of their underlying lung process when infected with influenza, and some studies have shown that the combination of the two can cause permanent loss of lung function.

Elderly Adults

In the elderly, fever is still a frequent finding but is more likely to be associated with confusion or lethargy. The respiratory complaints may not be identifiable in the older patient at all during the initial stage of infection, but secondary bacterial pneumonia is more likely to occur in this age group. Overall, the elderly are at the greatest risk for developing complications from influenza infection. Factors that contribute to more severe influenza infections in older adults include the following: (1) decreased compliance of the lungs; (2) deficits in respiratory muscle strength; (3) declining immune system function, especially at the cellular level; and (4) decreased antibody response to new antigens.

Annual vaccination is recommended for all elderly patients, particularly if they reside in a nursing home. Prophylactic use of an antiviral medication can provide additional protection against influenza when used in conjunction with vaccination.

Immunocompromised Patients

In patients whose immune system is compromised by disease or medications, the severity of symptoms may be worse when influenza infection occurs. There is also an increased risk of serious complications such as primary viral pneumonia or secondary bacterial pneumonia, leading to high rates of hospitalization, intensive care unit admission, and mortality. Transplant recipients can experience a high likelihood of graft dysfunction and rejection after influenza infection. Severely immunocompromised patients will shed influenza virus for weeks to months after infection.

Pregnant Women

As has already been discussed in Chapter 3, pregnant women suffered disproportionately during the influenza pandemic of 1918. Newer studies have shown an increasing incidence of hospitalizations in pregnant women during the influenza season for acute heart and lung issues; the risk of hospitalization increased with length of pregnancy and in those with high-risk medical conditions. The ACIP includes pregnant women in the high-priority group recommended for influenza vaccination.

5

Making the Diagnosis of Influenza

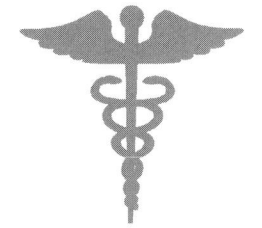

But nothing is more estimable than a physician who, having studied nature from his youth, knows the properties of the human body, the diseases which assail it, the remedies which benefit it, exercises his art with caution, and pays equal attention to the rich and the poor.

> François-Marie Arouet (known as Voltaire),
> French Philosopher and Writer

CLINICAL DIAGNOSIS OF INFLUENZA

With knowledge gleaned from medical study and clinical training, as well as that which comes with age and experience, a good medical practitioner should be able to identify the signs and symptoms suggestive of the diagnosis of influenza in an ill patient. The initial approach to a sick patient first involves attainment of a health history (often called the patient interview), which then is complemented by completion of a physical examination. The data compiled during the history and physical then guide the decisions regarding laboratory or radiology testing that might aid in achieving an accurate diagnosis.

Health History

A health history is essentially a story, told by the patient, about their current symptoms and their medical past. The history can vary with regard to detail and duration and is somewhat dependent on the age of the patient (and their ability to communicate to others). The health history is usually based on several core components, including the following:

Chief Complaint: Whenever possible, this complaint should be described and documented in the patient's own words. For example, a patient suffering from influenza might claim, "I felt great until this afternoon, when I began to suddenly feel feverish." If a patient is unable to verbalize their complaints directly (i.e., very young or very old patients), their caregivers might be able to explain what prompted them to seek medical attention for their ward.

History of Present Illness: This component of the history is simply a clear, chronological account of the symptoms that prompted the patient to seek medical attention. Good medical practitioners know that the main symptoms should be described in terms of the following:

1. location
2. quality
3. quantity or severity
4. timing
5. setting
6. factors or treatments that have either aggravated or relieved them
7. associated manifestations

In attempting to explain their troubles during a bout of influenza, a patient might note the following responses to the above inquiries about their primary symptoms:

1. "My symptoms are localized to the head, chest, and large muscle groups."
2. "I have fever, headache, a stuffy nose, a cough with greenish colored sputum, and aches in my back and calf muscles."
3. "The headache is pretty severe, and I feel worse when my fever is at its highest."
4. "I began to feel sick rather abruptly about two days ago, and the symptoms started about three days after I returned home from a trip by airplane."

5. "I have had some transient relief of symptoms with over-the-counter analgesics and cold medications. My fever is worse in the late afternoon and evening but seems to get better after I take acetaminophen."
6. "I also have started to notice that I don't have much of an appetite, and that I am really, really tired. It was hard to get myself out of bed this morning to keep this appointment."

Past Medical History: A patient's past health problems (including significant childhood illnesses), hospitalizations, accidents, and injuries should be reviewed. In pediatric patients, it is important to consider the birth history, developmental history, mother's health history, and immunizations as well. Conditions such as chronic lung disease or HIV positivity may predispose a patient to more severe illness when infected with influenza.

Past Surgical History: Previous procedures and operations are described in this section of the history.

Allergies: Primarily, this component of the history attempts to document the patient's allergies to medications. However, it is also important to document food and environmental allergies. In the interview of a patient with influenza, it is important to note any previous reactions to antiviral medications, vaccinations, or foods such as eggs; the presence of these could preclude use of either the antiviral medications or the influenza vaccination.

Medications: A complete list of the patient's medications should be reviewed, including home remedies, nonprescription and prescription drugs, vitamin and mineral supplements, and alternative therapies. Luckily, the antiviral medications used to treat, or prevent, influenza tend to have little in the way of drug interactions or contraindications.

Family History: The age and health status (or cause of death) of each immediate family member is helpful to know, particularly when considering a contagious disease such as influenza.

Social History: This component of the history is meant to capture the important psychosocial and behavioral information about a patient. Pertinent concerns include job history, marriage status, home situation, tobacco use, alcohol use, illicit drug use, religious beliefs, and military service.

Review of Systems: A full review of the systems of the body with regard to symptoms completes the history and often allows discovery of clues to a diagnosis that might not have been offered in the patient's own voice during the story of their present illness. Systems to consider include the following:

- general health
- skin

- head, eyes, ears, nose, and throat
- neck
- pulmonary (lungs)
- cardiac (heart)
- gastrointestinal
- genitourinary and breast
- musculoskeletal
- neurologic
- psychiatric

Interestingly, there are techniques to the patient interview that are taught to medical practitioners during their training that help in gathering accurate information in an efficient but empathetic manner. One such technique is to begin the interview with general, open-ended questions. This allows the full freedom of response and gives the patient a chance to tell their story. For example, a question such as "What brings you into the office to see me today?" prompts a much different response than a question such as "I understand you have a fever?" Once the patient has completed their story, more directed questions may then be appropriate to help clarify specific details about the patient's complaints. A medical practitioner must take care, however, not to ask what are known as leading questions. A patient who says "no" to the question "Does your sputum look purulent?" might not understand exactly what the practitioner meant by the description (purulent is a term that implies pus, a substance associated with infection). A better way to ask the question would be "Do you produce any sputum when you cough, and, if so, what does it look like?" It is also to the benefit of the practitioner to withhold interruptions during the patient interview. Medical studies have confirmed that physicians are quick to interrupt their patients during the explanation of their illness (one medical study has shown that physicians, on average, listen to their patients' concerns for about eighteen seconds before interrupting). It is now stressed during medical training that a more accurate history and, therefore, a better chance at accurate diagnosis, is likely if a patient can complete the story in their own words (on average, a patient will take two and a half minutes to tell their story completely, without interruption). Another technique used by medical practitioners is to ask questions that require a graded response rather than only a "yes" or "no" answer. For instance, the response to the question "How far can you walk before you must stop for breath?" will be different from "Do you get short of breath when you walk?" Also, it is important for the practitioner to ask one question at a time, in language that is understandable to the patient. A patient who answered "no" to the question "Do you have a history

Patient Etiquette for the Health History

Although they may not realize it, patients can also help their practitioners perform an efficient and accurate health history by considering the following recommendations:

- Spend time before the appointment formulating concerns. For example, a patient with influenza and worsening respiratory symptoms might want reassurance that the process has not led to a secondary bacterial pneumonia that would necessitate antibiotics, and may desire a prescription for medication to ease pain in the muscles and joints.
- Limit the list of concerns to a reasonable number (two or three, at most) and, if there are more issues that cannot be addressed during one appointment time slot, make another scheduled visit to finish the evaluation.
- Report concerns in a concise, clear manner and answer questions truthfully.
- Display a positive attitude and consider asking the practitioner, "What can I do to help myself feel better?"
- Avoid comments that might signal a sense of distrust, and try not to criticize other doctors or medical personnel. For instance, imagine a patient with influenza, diagnosed at the emergency room, who appropriately did not receive a prescription for antibiotics despite an insistence to be treated (remember, antibiotics do not work against a viral infection). The patient schedules an appointment with their general practitioner the next morning for follow-up, and again insists on antibiotic treatment while voicing opinions about the inadequacy of care at the emergency room. The patient is not more likely to receive (inappropriate) antibiotics from their astute practitioner, and they may have further compromised the doctor-patient relationship with an unnecessary visit, an unreasonable request for medications, and unwanted criticisms of potentially respected medical colleagues.
- Do not attempt to influence the practitioner's diagnosis or treatment with use of anecdotal experiences about other patients or doctors (conversely, do not withhold information about important sick contacts).
- Think about what a practitioner is expected to do with outside information brought to the visit from the library, the television, or the Internet (for example, clarification of the information, consideration for other treatments, or referral to a new practitioner or specialist).
- Try not to expect the impossible and keep expectations realistic. Influenza is not a "curable" infection, but a practitioner might be able to suggest some supportive treatments that will make a patient feel better until the disease process is over.
- Do not ask the practitioner to do something unethical or illegal.

of influenza, tuberculosis, pleurisy, pneumonia, or bronchitis?" might have had difficulty following the list of described illnesses or recognizing the terminology used. Finally, a good practitioner will always ask the patient, "Is there anything else you'd like to tell me?" before completing the interview.

The degree of detail needed for a health history is, in part, dictated by the complaints voiced by patient but also by the healthcare setting. It is obvious that a ten-minute appointment in a primary care clinic for acute onset of influenza necessitates a shorter, more targeted history than presentation to an emergency department at a hospital because of worsening respiratory complaints and concern for pneumonia. Regardless, once the history has been obtained, the healthcare provider often has a list of possible diagnoses already in mind; this list is called the differential diagnosis. The practitioner then moves on to the physical examination to look for additional clues that may aid in narrowing the differential to one unifying diagnosis that can then be targeted with treatment.

Physical Examination

With regard to the physical examination of a patient, a skillful practitioner is thorough yet efficient, systematic without rigidity, and gentle but competent. As with the patient interview, the completeness of the physical examination depends on the complaints, the healthcare setting, and the results of the health history. A targeted examination of the respiratory system may be enough to make the diagnosis of influenza in an urgent care clinic, but additional investigation of the body would be warranted for a patient that presents to the hospital with influenza complicated by heart failure or encephalitis.

A comprehensive physical examination begins with review of a patient's vital signs, which may include temperature, heart rate, respiratory rate, blood pressure, and weight. In the case of the patient with influenza, the temperature is often elevated, indicating fever. The heart rate and respiratory rate might also be increased as a response to the patient's fever, caused by the body's systemic reaction to infection. Blood pressure readings may be either high or low in the setting of active infection. Patients may also note weight loss during a bout of influenza, particularly if bothered by gastrointestinal symptoms. The remaining components of a full physical exam might include the following:

- General survey: The patient's mental status, level of consciousness, posture, and odor should be observed. The patient's overall appearance should be documented, particularly whether they appear "toxic" or whether they are in pain or distress. Patients suffering from influenza can look quite ill (particularly during spikes in fever), even when the disease is uncomplicated. They may appear tired, and older patients might even seem somewhat confused.

- Skin: Any rash or lesions should be noted. Influenza can also cause sweats, flushing of the skin, and warmth attributable to fever. In severe cases, cyanosis (a bluish, cold tinge to the skin caused by poor oxygen exchange) can be seen, particularly at the lips and fingertips.
- Head, eyes, ears, nose, and throat: It is not unusual for influenza infection to cause watery eyes, injection of the conjunctiva, burning of the eyes, nasal congestion, rhinorrhea, and pharyngitis. On examination, a practitioner might notice tears, red eyes, a stuffed or runny nose, or inflamed nasal passages and throat. The patient's voice might also be hoarse.
- Neck: The neck should be palpated at the front and back. Enlarged lymph nodes might be appreciated in influenza patients, and these can be tender to the touch (particularly in children).
- Pulmonary: Auscultation of the lungs from both the anterior and posterior aspects is important in looking for abnormalities that can be seen in influenza infection. The practitioner may notice that the air "crackles" as it travels through congested airways, and the patient may cough during the evaluation. Some patients might have chest pain, or pleurisy, when taking deep breaths during their evaluation. Pneumonia can also be suspected if palpation or percussion of the thorax reveals abnormalities.
- Cardiovascular: As noted above, the heart rate is often elevated in patients in the midst of a bout of the flu. Occasionally, an alert practitioner can detect subtle abnormalities in the heart rhythm that can be caused by infection with influenza.
- Gastrointestinal: Practitioners will usually auscultate and palpate the abdomen, which can be tender in some patients with the flu (especially if they have had nausea and vomiting that have strained their abdominal muscles). Enlargement of the liver and spleen is not normally found in influenza.
- Musculoskeletal: Myalgias (muscle aches) and arthralgias (joint pain) can be documented during the examination of influenza patients, and joints can be stiff or swollen.
- Neurologic: Occasionally, influenza can be complicated by central nervous system involvement, leading to neurological deficits that can be appreciated on physical examination. The findings of confusion, lethargy, stupor, or even varying degrees of paralysis may be documented.

Patient Etiquette for the Physical Examination

A patient can aid their practitioner in completing an efficient but accurate physical examination by remembering a few key concepts:

- In current medical practice, it is not unusual for a practitioner to wear gloves during the entire examination. The gloves are not meant to alienate or isolate the patient and are often used as part of a universal precautionary protocol.
- Try not to voice a list of important concerns during the examination itself. It is tempting to talk while the practitioner is quiet, but they are often concentrating or using the stethoscope during such moments.
- If a patient would like their practitioner to explain each part of the examination while it is being performed, ask in advance rather than while the exam is being conducted. A practitioner is less likely to tell an influenza patient what was heard on the lung evaluation if a patient asks about the findings while the stethoscope is still in place.
- Do not be surprised if a practitioner asks additional questions during certain parts of the examination. These questions do not necessarily imply that the doctor has found something of concern but may rather be a supplement to the earlier health history. For example, during the abdominal exam, a doctor may ask an influenza patient if they have had trouble with nausea or vomiting if it was not voiced as a concern initially.
- A patient should feel comfortable with asking questions about the findings when the physician has finished the examination.

Other Considerations

Another helpful piece of information for practitioners as they attempt to make the diagnosis of influenza in their patients is knowledge of the virus' activity in the region. When the presence of influenza has been confirmed in a community, most patients who present with a flu-like illness will truly have the flu. The accuracy of the clinical diagnosis alone, without any complementary laboratory or radiology testing, in the midst of an influenza outbreak can reach 80–90 percent.

Studies have attempted to identify parameters that might allow better prediction of the findings on the history and physical exam for the accurate diagnosis of influenza. A recently published systematic review of the medical literature with regard to use of the health history and physical examination to diagnose influenza identified three key variables: rigors (shaking chills), sweating, and fever, with onset of symptoms less than three days before

---

Testing Patients for Avian Influenza

In some circumstances, it may be necessary to consider testing a patient specifically for avian influenza.

- Patients who are considered high risk for avian influenza and require testing include those who have a history of travel to a country with documented H5N1 in poultry and/or humans within ten days of the start of symptoms and pneumonia confirmed by X-ray, ARDS, or other severe respiratory illness for which another cause has not been found.
- Low-risk patients are those with a history of contact with domestic poultry (or a suspected human case) in a country with H5N1 within ten days of the start of symptoms and fever of at least 38 degrees Celsius and one or more of the following symptoms: cough, sore throat, or shortness of breath. These patients should also be considered for specific avian influenza testing.

---

presentation. Additional features that would argue against influenza as a diagnosis include a lack of systemic complaints, no report of cough, being able to cope with daily activities, and not being confined to bed. Another published study evaluated patients over the age of sixty-five or patients with an underlying cardiopulmonary disease, who were admitted to the hospital with a respiratory diagnosis. Twenty percent of these patients were found to have influenza. The best predictor of an accurate diagnosis of influenza in this study was a combination of cough, a temperature of thirty-eight degrees Celsius or higher, and a duration of symptoms of seven days or less.

Occasionally, use of an imaging study may also help in the diagnosis of influenza. An X-ray of the chest may show abnormalities consistent with primary viral pneumonia or secondary bacterial pneumonia. Computed tomography of the thorax, allowing a three-dimensional picture, can reveal additional complications in the lung and pleural space.

LABORATORY DIAGNOSIS OF INFLUENZA

Even with the skill of a wise practitioner, establishing a diagnosis of influenza purely based on clinical symptoms can sometimes be difficult. Other respiratory illnesses caused by a variety of infectious agents can mimic the symptoms of influenza, and the reported sensitivity of diagnosing influenza accurately based solely on symptoms varies greatly. Using laboratory tests to confirm the diagnosis of influenza if it is suspected by the findings of the health history and physical examination can lead to more appropriate treatment recommendations. The laboratory diagnosis of influenza is also important in helping to prevent, contain, monitor, and treat the illness. Now, with the concern for an emerging, highly pathogenic avian influenza virus that might lead to a worldwide pandemic, the ability to use the laboratory to isolate and subtype the virus to aid in epidemiological surveillance and production of a vaccine becomes even more significant.

Historically, laboratory testing for influenza has not been considered to be of much value to the common health practitioner because the turnaround time for laboratory testing did not provide a diagnosis in the acute setting, the tests available were not highly sensitive for influenza, and there were little treatment options to offer even if the diagnosis could be confirmed. Now, however, the development of more rapid and accurate tests for the detection of influenza provides clinicians with a way to confirm a prompt and accurate diagnosis of the disease. In turn, this has allowed more timely initiation of antiviral therapies, avoidance of injudicious use of antibiotics, implementation of appropriate infection control and containment measures, decreased need and duration of hospitalization, reduction in unnecessary ancillary laboratory or radiology testing, and, overall, decreased healthcare costs.

Current laboratory techniques can attempt to detect either the virus itself or the patient's immune response to the virus.

Viral Culture

Although the flow of mucus from the nose or the production of phlegm from a cough might be uncomfortable for the sick patient, it actually provides a practitioner the means by which to make a diagnosis. In the case of influenza, a swab from the nose or throat, washings taken from nasal passages, or a collection of sputum produced by cough can provide a sample of fluid that can be tested for the virus. Once expressed from the patient, the samples are put into special vials of viral transport medium and sent to the laboratory for analysis in a timely manner. Luckily, the influenza virus can live overnight in the proper specimen container if it is kept on ice.

Of all of the specimen types, the throat swab is the least likely to yield a positive culture; the other specimens have a tendency for higher yield. More than 90 percent of positive cultures can be detected within three days of inoculation, and the remainder by five to seven days. Obviously, the time required for a culture to turn positive is the downside to such testing: by the time the diagnosis is made by growth of the virus on culture medium, a patient could be either in recovery or, unfortunately in the case of pandemic influenza, potentially even dead.

False-negative tests can occur because of several reasons, including (1) low quantities of the viral particle in some respiratory samples; (2) inappropriately collected, handled, and/or transported specimens; (3) the presence of viral inhibitors; and (4) the emergence of new viral subtypes for which the tests are not designed. False-positive laboratory findings can also occur, and factors contributing to this inaccurate diagnosis include (1) laboratory error (either clerical or operational) and (2) suboptimal design of the test in question.

There are two types of viral culture techniques for influenza:

- Conventional culture: This technique originally involved inoculation of patient specimens into the amniotic cavity of ten- to twelve-day-old embryonated chicken eggs. Although able to provide high yields of virus after three days of incubation, this process is now primarily used only in reference laboratories (see Figure 5.1). Newer techniques for culture require inoculation of the patient's specimen into prepared single layers of cell cultures; these are then monitored for the development of cytopathic effects (pathological changes in the appearance of the cells), for manifestation of hemadsorption (the adherence of red blood cells to other surfaces) after the addition of erythrocytes, or for the presence of influenza antigen by specific antibody staining.
- Rapid shell vial culture: This technique uses a prepared single or mixed cell line but enhances the viral infectivity of the cells by centrifugation. This process provides a better chance of accurate positive testing, as well as a shortened time to detection (twenty-four hours compared with three or more days with the conventional culture technique).

Rapid Antigen Tests

Luckily, more rapid testing measures than cultures for influenza are now available and are based on an immunologic concept: the detection of viral antigen in respiratory secretions by interaction with a specific antibody. In the easy-to-use, self-contained, rapid antigen tests, a sample of respiratory secretions is treated with an agent to break apart mucus and then tested, on a filter paper, in an optical device, or with a dipstick, for a color change reaction that signifies the binding of an antibody to an influenza antigen. In a somewhat similar manner, another type of rapid antigen test detects the presence of viral NA activity in the patient's sample by using a pigmented substrate. The rapid antigen tests are designed to detect both influenza A and influenza B strains of virus, are fairly simple to perform in the laboratory, and can provide results within sixty minutes.

If the patient sample of respiratory secretions was obtained with accuracy and care, the tests can report a true positive result about 40–80 percent of the time. The test occasionally shows negative when the disease is actually present (0–15 percent of the time). The tests are most accurate in young children simply because the children shed much larger quantities of virus in their respiratory secretions. This is also true for older patients early in their illness, when shedding is highest. These tests are most likely to be successful if performed on nasopharyngeal aspirates, more so than on nasopharyngeal swabs, or throat swabs or gargles. Because of variety in the sampling techniques and the range in sensitivity and specificity of these rapid antigen techniques, it is preferable that providers have access to a reference laboratory to resolve any unclear test results. It has been shown that, when used at the point of care (for example, at a doctor's

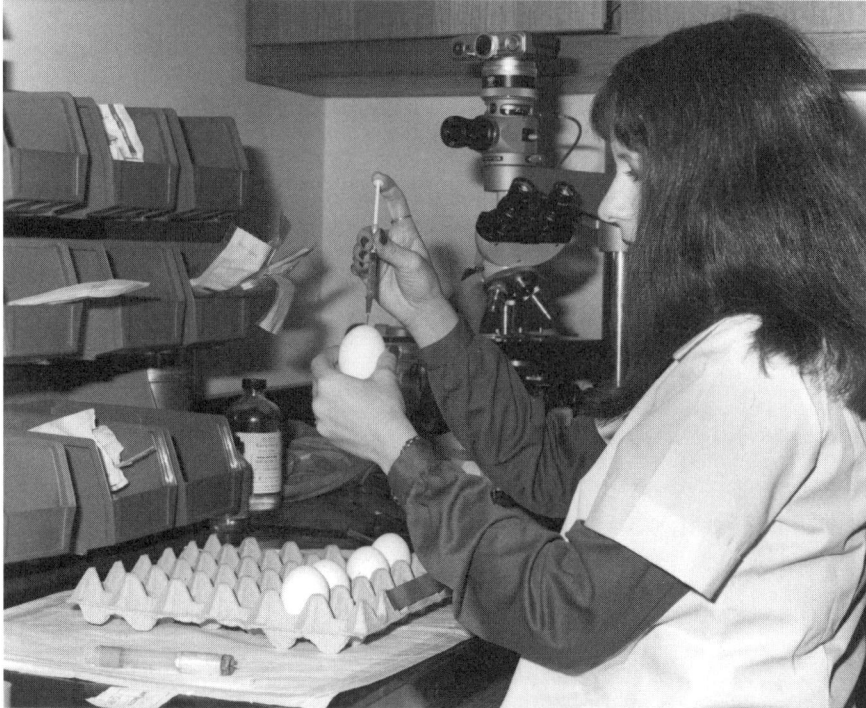

Figure 5.1. Inoculation of Embryonic Chicken Eggs. A photograph, dated 1968, of a CDC laboratorian inoculating 10-day old embryonated chicken eggs with specimens containing the influenza virus. Image used with permission, courtesy of the CDC.

office or urgent care clinic), the rapid antigen tests lead to reduced patient costs by limiting the use of inappropriate antibiotics, decreasing orders for blood cultures, and allowing avoidance of unnecessary chest X-rays.

Immunofluorescence Microscopy

Also known as a direct fluorescent antibody test or an immunofluorescent antibody test, this method involves staining of respiratory epithelial cells with specific antibodies, which are linked to a fluorescent dye. The accuracy of these tests depends on the presence of an adequate number of infected cells and can vary according to the specimen type submitted for analysis.

Nucleic Acid Testing

Another approach to testing for influenza is by amplification of the viral genetic sequences by reverse-transcription PCR or nucleic acid sequence-based amplification. These are sensitive tests and can even allow the diagnosis of influenza in tissues or specimens in which the virus has lost its viability. These tests are not yet in common use because they are more labor intensive, are technically demanding, require special equipment, and are potentially more expensive to perform; however, they are replacing viral isolation and culture as the reference standard. Another benefit to these tests is that they can more readily identify influenza viruses in immunosuppressed transplant patients and in persons with chronic lung diseases (these patient groups have been hard to test in the past because of low levels of virus along the respiratory tract despite obvious symptomatic illness). The ability to accurately diagnose and treat this particular patient group is crucial if a healthcare provider is to decrease an individual patient's risk of morbidity and mortality and to prevent further spread of infection (particularly in a healthcare setting).

Serological Testing

Once the illness caused by influenza is over, the chance of making a diagnosis by clinical evaluation or by rapid antigen testing is low. Instead, by obtaining paired blood samples from patients, a rise in antibody levels can be detected over time, implying that infection with influenza has occurred. The first specimen is drawn within two weeks of illness (known as the acute phase), followed by a second sample several weeks later (called the convalescent phase). A single specimen is not particularly helpful because most people have been exposed to influenza at some point during their lifetime and have a baseline level of antibody that can be detected. A fourfold or more rise in the influenza antibody levels noted between the acute phase and convalescent phase of illness is diagnostic of infection. In addition, serological testing can be used to measure the response to influenza vaccination, because there should be a rise in antibody after the vaccine has been administered. Of note, there are four main types of serological tests available for the diagnosis of influenza: (1) virus neutralization, (2) HA inhibition assays, (3) complement fixation, and (4) enzyme immunoassay tests.

Additional Laboratory Considerations

Along with testing that allows confirmation of the influenza diagnosis either by identification of the virus itself or by measurement of the host's immune system response to infection, other laboratory evaluation may give clues to a patient's diagnosis of influenza, particularly if the clinical course is complicated. Blood tests can be performed to look for an elevated white blood cell reaction, which is often an indicator of infection or stress. Blood cultures specifically for bacteria or fungi can ensure that there is not an alternative pathogen responsible for a patient's symptoms. Analysis of oxygen exchange in the blood can verify concerns for severe pulmonary involvement and can confirm suspicions of cyanosis seen on clinical evaluation. Spinal fluid analysis can reveal reaction to the virus in the central nervous system. Liver enzyme testing can be a clue to the occurrence of Reye's syndrome. Usually, such ancillary testing is unnecessary because the diagnosis of the flu is often made by clinical assessment and specific influenza testing, but decisions regarding additional laboratory analysis should be guided by the clinician's initial health history and physical examination results.

FUTURE DEVELOPMENT OF DIAGNOSTIC TESTS FOR INFLUENZA

The current laboratory diagnostic options are fairly effective for testing during seasonal influenza outbreaks and even for sporadic epidemics of the virus. However, new developments are in progress to enhance diagnostic capabilities, particularly for testing in prepandemic and pandemic scenarios. Several new technologies are based on amplification of the nucleic acids found in the viral genome after hybridization to target probes, followed by monitoring with an automated reader. It is also expected that other new developments will include more sensitive and more specific rapid antigen tests to be performed at the point of care, and the use of expanded nucleic acid testing that would provide same-day results in larger laboratory settings.

6

Treatment and Prevention of Influenza

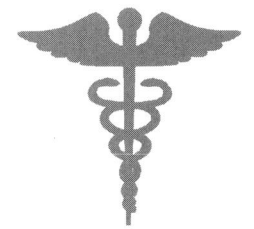

In my experience much depends upon the promptness and thoroughness of the treatment prosecuted within the first twenty-four hours. Two or three thorough early treatments will certainly prove very effective. Also, if possible, have the patient take an eight-minute hot bath, a hot lemonade and wrap himself in a blanket for twenty or twenty-five minutes until he perspires freely. Clean out the bowels with an enema; there is usually moderate constipation. Keep patient in bed until temperature returns to normal and has been normal for a day or two. Avoid chilling. A warm room freely ventilated is best in my opinion. Sponge baths are beneficial and soothing. Give a reasonable amount of fluids, and do not restrict the food unduly. Hot fomentations over the aching parts, such as neck, dorsal and sacral regions will give considerable relief. The osteopathic manipulative therapy is of great value, but care has to be taken that it is correctly and carefully performed. Rough and prolonged treatment is strictly contraindicated.*

C. P. McConnell, D.O., October of 1918

As made clear in the above editorial by Dr. McConnell, published originally in the *Journal of the American Osteopathic Association* during the influenza pandemic of 1918 and reprinted in 2000, there has

*Used by permission of the American Osteopathic Association.

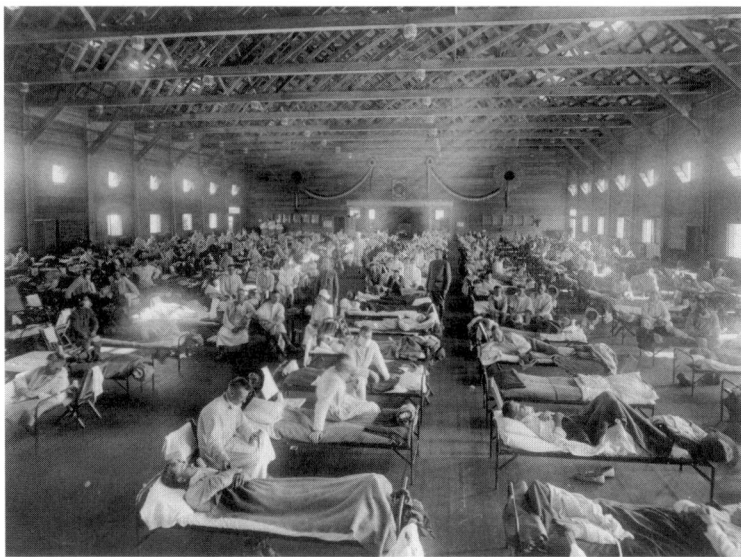

Figure 6.1. Emergency Hospital for Influenza Patients. An emergency hospital created to treat patients at Camp Furston in Kansas, 1918. Image used with permission from the 1918 Influenza Epidemic Gallery, courtesy of the National Museum of Health and Medicine, Armed Forces Institute of Pathology.

historically been little to offer people who became ill with the virus outside of supportive care. Both medical professionals and patients willingly tried "scientific" remedies and preventives suspected to be helpful. With the influenza virus not yet known to exist, the primary cause of concern was either spread of a bacteria or exposure to miasma (essentially something "foul" in the air). Physicians at the time proposed that patients might benefit from aggressive antiseptic cleansing of individual bodies and even public places. Community fountains were sterilized with blowtorches, and public telephones were wiped with alcohol. It was recommended that people not shake hands with one another upon greeting or parting, and that gauze masks be worn when they had to venture out of doors (this was even put into law in some communities). Teeth were pulled and tonsils removed in the hope that infection would be excised along with the body parts. Steam vapor mixed with eucalyptus or camphor was inhaled. Antitoxins and vaccines were produced and tried, and medicines used successfully for other diseases were prescribed (for example, sulfur was put in clothing). Schools, churches, and theaters were closed; quarantines were attempted. Emergency hospitals were created to help house the sick patients (see Figure 6.1). However, none of these remedies had a measurable effect, and it is now understood that none of them offered a true cure for influenza.

Luckily, identification of the influenza virus and further comprehension of its structure ultimately allowed research focusing on treatment alternatives to be performed, and both preventative and symptomatic relief therapies are now available. As of yet, however, a true cure for influenza still does not exist, and the virus continues to plague humankind in its seasonal outbreaks and its potential for spread of an impressive pandemic in the future.

TREATMENTS FOR INFLUENZA

Supportive Care

In many cases of influenza, bed rest, along with vigorous maintenance of hydration, often are the treatments of choice. Other considerations for supportive care include the following:

- Ingestion of acetylsalicyclic acid (aspirin) or other analgesic and antipyretic agents to combat headache, fever, and myalgias or athralgias. Note that use of aspirin must be avoided in children eighteen years or younger because of the association with Reye's syndrome.
- Use of sprays or drops to treat congestion and obstruction of the nasal passages. It should be noted that decongestant sprays can only be used for three consecutive days, or a phenomenon known as rebound congestion might occur (expansion of the tiny blood vessels in the nose, leading to feelings of congestion, which prompt a cycle of more and more use of the spray). If sneezing is also problematic, ingestion of a traditional antihistamine might be beneficial.
- Gargling with a saline mixture two or three times a day to relieve throat pain or hoarse voice.
- Use of suppressants to ease or alleviate cough. Liquid suppressants with dextromethorphan or codeine (this requires a prescription) often work well if used as directed by label instructions.
- Attention to nutrition, with light meals, ingestion of tea, a glass of orange juice daily, and avoidance of high-fat foods.
- Antibiotics for treatment of identified or suspected secondary bacterial infection.
- Fluid repletion with intravenous access may be necessary if dehydration occurs. Replacement of electrolytes (sodium, potassium, etc.) occasionally is warranted.
- Administration of oxygen and, in severe cases, consideration of intubation with use of mechanical ventilation to assist breathing.

In addition to supportive care measures, the benefits of infection control methods cannot be overemphasized. Simple acts such as proper hand hygiene, cough etiquette (for example, covering the mouth while coughing with hands or an upper arm), and avoidance of sick contacts could have a significant impact on decreasing the spread of influenza and limiting the likelihood of severe infection in at-risk patient populations.

Antiviral Drugs

There are four antiviral drugs currently available for prevention and/or treatment of influenza. It should be noted, however, that most individuals with an intact immune system who have previously been exposed to influenza (and thus have some "immune system memory" of the virus) often limit the replication of the virus rapidly on their own. Thus, the opportunity to influence viral replication with antiviral medications is somewhat limited, and effective use of the available remedies requires early initiation of the medications. No studies have ever demonstrated a benefit of antiviral therapy if they are started after symptoms have been present for forty-eight hours, and the greatest effect has been demonstrated when medications are started within the first twenty-four hours of becoming ill.

Because a cure of the virus is not possible with use of the currently available antiviral medications, some of the goals of treatment may be the following: (1) to treat ill patients with the hope of lessening the severity of disease and to treat those at high-risk for additional complications of the disease; (2) to provide prophylaxis for essential medical and governing personnel who might need to provide front-line care in the midst of an outbreak and to provide prophylaxis to exposed individuals, such as family members of already ill patients; (3) to treat the healthy with the hope of reducing the burden on the healthcare system and decreasing the spread of the virus; and (4) to abort the emergence of a new influenza A subtype.

Antiviral medications targeting influenza can be divided into two main categories: M2 inhibitors and neuraminidase inhibitors.

M2 Inhibitors

The influenza virus contains M proteins: the M1 protein is involved in the structural matrix of the virus, whereas the M2 protein is known to be an ion channel pump. This pump allows the interior of the influenza virus to maintain an appropriate balance of acidity, which is necessary for transport of the viral genome into the nucleus of a host cell; from there, the virus can proceed with replication. The drugs known as M2 inhibitors exert their effect on the influenza virus by limiting the workings of the ion channel pump mechanism, thereby influencing viral acidity and preventing viral "uncoating." If the virus cannot shed its outer coat as it is incorporated into the human host cell, it cannot proceed with replication. Without replication, the virus cannot make new particles to spread to and, consequently, infect other host cells. It is of interest to note that similar ion channels have been found in influenza B and C strains, but the M2 inhibitor medications do not appear to have any activity against these versions of influenza and can only be used for influenza A.

There are two drugs currently available in the M2 inhibitor category: amantadine and rimantadine. Both drugs are available as oral medications that can be ingested. Like the similarities in their names, these medications are related to each other in terms of their structures, and they are active against all strains of influenza A. There are a few notable differences between amantadine and rimantadine, however.

Both amantadine and rimantadine have proven to be effective against both experimentally induced and naturally occurring influenza A. Amantadine was studied extensively during the 1968 influenza pandemic with the viral strain H3N2. When ingested by patients within the first two days of illness, amantadine reduced the duration of fever by about twenty-four hours. Treated individuals also reported more rapid improvement in cough, sore throat, and nasal congestion. In the late 1970s, additional trials of amantadine therapy were performed with the H1N1 viral strain; similar results were reported. Treated adults showed a more rapid decrease in fever and improved symptoms at forty-eight hours when compared with subjects given a placebo. Treated subjects were also less likely to shed virus. Studies with rimantadine have showed similar success. Subjects treated with rimantadine during infection with H1N1 and H3N2 viral strains of influenza A had improved symptoms, decreased fever, and reduced viral shedding when compared with individuals given a placebo. Rimantadine has also been studied in children and reduces the level of viral shedding early in infection. However, rimantadine is not currently licensed for treatment of children in the United States. Direct comparison of amantadine with rimantadine has shown no difference in efficacy.

Unfortunately, drug resistance has been a factor in limiting the more widespread use of the M2 inhibitors. Up until 2003, reported resistance of the influenza virus for either amantadine or rimantadine was rare, but it has unfortunately increased in frequency since that time. Resistant viruses are not usually seen in individuals who have not previously been exposed to the antiviral medications. However, they emerge fairly frequently in treated individuals, particularly children. Resistance is usually the result of mutations in the M2 protein itself, and, once the necessary mutation(s) are present, resistance is conferred to both drugs in the M2 inhibitor category. Because of the risk of emergence of resistance during treatment, the drugs are not recommended for use during an actual epidemic. For now, both amantadine and rimantadine have been removed from the CDC list of recommended medications for treatment of influenza A in the United States and will likely not be therapeutic alternatives until evidence of susceptibility has been reestablished among circulating influenza A viral strains.

Amantadine (trade name Symmetrel) is a stable white crystalline powder, freely soluble in water and soluble in alcohol and in chloroform, and is made available to patients as 100 mg capsules. For treatment of influenza, the usual adult daily dosage is 200 mg, taken as two 100 mg capsules as a single daily dose, or split into one capsule of 100 mg twice a day. For elderly individuals (age sixty-five years or older), the daily dosage is decreased to 100 mg. For pediatric patients between one and nine years of age, the total daily dose is calculated on the basis of weight: 2–4 mg/lb/day (4.4–8.8 mg/kg/day); the total dose should not exceed 150 mg/day. For children nine to twelve years of age, the total daily dose is 200 mg given as one capsule of 100 mg twice a day.

Amantadine, unlike rimantadine, does not undergo metabolic change during intake into the human body and is eventually excreted unchanged in the urine. This is an important distinction to remember when considering an individual patient's health status, particularly those with kidney failure and the elderly (who inherently may have decreased kidney function attributable to age). In both of these patient groups, the excretion of amantadine into the urine can be considerably slowed. If the drug cannot be excreted normally, it instead accumulates rapidly in the body and causes unwanted side effects. Thus, it is of interest to adjust the dosage of amantadine in these patient populations to avoid toxic consequences, and a dosage decrease to 100 mg daily is recommended.

The side effects that can occur with use of amantadine are usually minor, and most frequently are reported as nausea, dizziness or lightheadedness, and insomnia. During initial studies with amantadine, side effects were carefully monitored and recorded with regard to frequency and ultimately divided into distinct categories, as shown in Table 6.1.

Once amantadine was made available to the general public, additional reports of side effects were documented:

- nervous system or psychiatric: coma, stupor, delirium, slowed movement, increased tone, delusions, aggressive behavior, paranoid reaction, manic reaction, involuntary muscle contractions, gait abnormalities, sensory alterations, electroencephalogram changes, and tremor

Table 6.1.
Side Effects of Amantadine

Frequency of side effects (percentage of patients)	Description of side effects (reported by patients)
5–10%	Nausea, dizziness (or lightheadedness), and insomnia
1–5%	Depression, anxiety and irritability, hallucinations, confusion, lack of appetite, dry mouth, constipation, abnormal balance or movement, livedo reticularis, peripheral edema, orthostatic hypotension, headache, somnolence, nervousness, dream abnormality, agitation, dry nose, diarrhea, fatigue
0.1–1%	Congestive heart failure, psychosis, urinary retention, difficulty breathing, skin rash, vomiting, weakness, slurred speech, euphoria, thinking abnormality, amnesia, hyperkinesias, hypertension, decreased libido, visual disturbance, including punctate subepithelial or other corneal opacity, corneal edema, decreased visual acuity, sensitivity to light, optic nerve palsy
Less than 0.1%	Convulsions, leukopenia, neutropenia, eczematoid determatitis, oculogyric episodes, suicidal attempt, suicide, suicidal ideation

- cardiovascular: cardiac arrest, abnormal heart rhythms, low blood pressure, and elevated heart rate
- respiratory: acute respiratory failure, pulmonary edema, and increased rate of breathing
- gastrointestinal: difficulty swallowing and painful swallow
- hematologic: leukocytosis and lack of white blood cell production
- special senses: inflamed eyes and abnormal dilation of the pupils
- skin and appendages: itching and sweating
- miscellaneous: neuroleptic malignant syndrome and allergic reactions, including anaphylactic reactions, edema, and fever
- laboratory tests: elevated muscle enzymes, kidney markers, serum, bilirubin, and liver enzymes

Treatment of influenza with amantadine should be started as soon as possible after appreciation of symptoms. Preferably, a sick patient should initiate the medication within twenty-four to forty-eight hours after recognizing that they may be ill with the flu, and amantadine should be continued for twenty-four to forty-eight hours after the disappearance of signs and symptoms.

Rimantadine (trade name Flumadine) is also a white to off-white crystalline powder that is freely soluble in water. It is available for oral ingestion as a

100 mg film-coated tablet and as a syrup solution. For treatment of influenza, the recommended adult dose of rimantadine is 100 mg twice a day. Rimantadine, compared with amantadine, undergoes extensive metabolism after ingestion into the human body, and less than 15 percent of the drug is excreted in the urine unchanged. Although this implies that patients with kidney failure attributable to age or disease are less likely to have difficulty with side effects of the medication, some patients have still demonstrated a tendency toward adverse effects; dosage reduction to 100 mg/day is recommended in elderly or nursing home patients and in those patients with severe hepatic dysfunction or renal failure. Rimantadine tends to cause less side effects related to the central nervous system than amantadine, and there are no known drug interactions with other medications.

During initial studies with rimantadine, side effects were carefully monitored and recorded, as noted in Table 6.2.

For influenza treatment, rimantadine therapy should be initiated as soon as possible, preferably within 48 hours after onset of signs and symptoms. Therapy should be continued for approximately seven days from the initial onset of symptoms.

Neuraminidase Inhibitors

Oseltamivir and zanamivir belong to the second category of antiviral agents that provide activity against influenza: the neuraminidase inhibitors. Both

Table 6.2.
Side Effects of Rimantadine

Frequency of side effects (percentage of patients)	Description of side effects (reported by patients)
1–3%	Insomnia, dizziness, headache, nervousness, fatigue, nausea, vomiting, anorexia, dry mouth, abdominal pain, asthenia
0.3–1%	Diarrhea, dyspepsia, impairment of concentration, ataxia, somnolence, agitation, depression, rash, tinnitus, difficulty breathing
Less than 0.3%	Gait abnormality, euphoria, hyperkinesia, tremor, hallucination, confusion, convulsions, bronchospasm, cough, pallor, palpitation, hypertension, cerebrovascular disorder, cardiac failure, pedal edema, heart block, tachycardia, syncope, non-puerperal lactation, taste loss/change, abnormal sense of smell

drugs work by inhibiting the function of the influenza virus' neuraminidase inhibitors. NA appears to be necessary for full penetration of the influenza virus into a host cell and for separation of a newly created viral particle. Without a functional NA molecule, the virus remains connected to the host cell and cannot perpetuate its disease process.

Luckily, oseltamivir and zanamivir work against both influenza A and influenza B, although they work more strongly against A strains. Avian viruses with all nine known NA subtypes appear to be sensitive to both drugs, as well. In early experimental studies, oseltamivir, given a day after onset of infection, resulted in reduction in viral shedding, reduced symptoms reported by patients, and decreased frequencies of middle ear abnormalities when compared with placebo. Zanamivir, given as late as fifty hours after infection, also demonstrated efficacy with subjects showing reduced viral shedding, decreased symptom scores, decreased nasal mucus weights, and less middle ear abnormalities.

Similar benefits were seen when both agents were tested in patients with uncomplicated influenza. Therapy with oseltamivir initiated within the first thirty-six hours of symptoms resulted in 30–40 percent reduction in the duration of symptoms and severity of illness, as well as reduced rates of prolonged coughing. Early administration of the drug was also associated with a significantly earlier return to work or other normal activities. Zanamivir, when given early in the course of symptoms to adults with either uncomplicated influenza A or B, also showed reduction in the duration of symptoms and an earlier return to normal activities. Early administration of zanamivir may also reduce the frequency of complications, with reductions in the use of antibacterial medications and in hospitalization.

Historically, resistance has not been a major issue for the neuraminidase inhibitors. Unfortunately, however, a small increase in the number of influenza viruses resistant to oseltamivir has been observed in the United States (5.7 percent of the 471 influenza A and B viruses tested thus far) during the 2007–2008 season. This is appreciably more than the 0.7 percent found to be resistant during the 2006–2007 season. All of the resistance has been documented in H1N1 strains of influenza A; no resistance has been found in H3N2 strains or in any influenza B subtypes. Naturally occurring viral resistance to zanamivir is not known to exist, and none of the viral strains tested in 2007–2008 have shown zanamivir resistance. Monitoring for the development of additional resistance after clinical use of the drugs will need to be done. One study has suggested that children may have a higher incidence of resistance development, with nine of fifty (18 percent) children taking oseltamivir showing evidence of viral strains with NA mutations.

Known by the trade name Tamiflu, oseltamivir is a white crystalline solid available to patients as capsules for ingestion or as a powder for oral suspension when reconstituted with water. It is approved for the treatment of influenza in persons one year and older. It is rapidly absorbed from the gastrointestinal tract as a prodrug and then converted in the liver to an active drug. The active drug is excreted in the urine unchanged. Adult dosing is recommended (for those aged thirteen and over) at 75 mg twice daily for five days. Dosage adjustment is recommended for patients with reduced kidney function to 75 mg given once daily for five days. Oseltamivir has been associated with transient gastrointestinal side effects, such as nausea and vomiting. Rarely, serious skin and hypersensitivity reactions have occurred; patients who have developed a rash or allergic symptoms while taking oseltamivir should alert their healthcare provider immediately of their findings. Use of probenecid at the same time as oseltamivir can cause competitive inhibition of excretion by the renal tubular epithelial cell anionic transporter; this can cause double the exposure to oseltamivir and could cause unwanted toxicities or side effects.

Although oseltamivir and zanamivir are both in the same category of antiviral medications, only oseltamivir is licensed for use in children. Although not recommended for patients who are less than twelve months of age, the dosing for pediatric patients one year and older is weight based: 2.5 mL (one half a teaspoon) for children weighing 15 kg or less, 3.8 mL (three quarters teaspoon) for children weighing more than 15–23 kg, 5.0 mL (one teaspoon) for children weighing 24–40 kg, and 6.2 mL (one and one quarter teaspoon) for children weighing more than 40 kg. In the pediatric population, the drug has been shown to be well tolerated with few worrisome side effects. It has also been associated with a reduction in symptom duration, as well as a 44 percent reduction in the frequency of otitis media (middle ear) complications.

Zanamivir (trade name Relenza) is supplied as a dry power for oral inhalation; it cannot be swallowed in pill or solution form. The drug is excreted unchanged in the urine, with full excretion of a single dose completed within a twenty-four-hour period. The recommended dose of zanamivir for the treatment of influenza in adults and children aged seven years and older is 10 mg twice daily (two consecutive inhalations of a 5 mg blister) for five days. On the first day of treatment, two doses should be taken at least two hours apart. On the following days, doses should be taken about twelve hours apart. There is no dosage adjustment in patients with renal impairment. However, patients with underlying pulmonary disease should always have a fast-acting bronchodilator available and should discontinue zanamivir if any respiratory difficulty develops during use.

During early studies in adult patients with use of zanamivir, some side effects and adverse events were documented. With rare occurrence, patients with asthma or chronic obstructive pulmonary disease had exacerbation of their pulmonary symptoms with bronchospasm and wheezing. Some additional side effects and adverse events were documented or observed during subsequent clinical use of zanamivir, as follows:

- allergic reactions: facial or oropharyngeal edema, itching, pain, redness, swelling or watering of eye or eyelid, troubled breathing or wheezing, severe skin rash or hives, flushing, increased sensitivity to sunlight, joint pain, swollen glands, and tightness in throat
- ear, nose, and throat: nasal signs and symptoms, change in hearing, earache, pain in ear, ear drainage, and pain and pressure over the cheeks
- cardiac: dizziness, fainting, and fast, slow, or irregular heartbeat
- pulmonary: difficulty breathing, shortness of breath, tightness in chest or wheezing, and cough with mucus production
- central nervous system: convulsions and headache
- gastrointestinal: diarrhea, nausea, and vomiting

PREVENTION OF INFLUENZA

Influenza Vaccines

As stated in the Recommendations of the ACIP for the Prevention and Control of Influenza in 2007, influenza vaccination is the most effective method for preventing infection and its potentially severe complications. To understand why this statement is given with such authority, knowledge of the scientific concepts behind vaccination, and its development through history, is necessary.

Another disease attributable to a virus that has resulted in great devastation in human history is smallpox, caused by the infectious agent named variola (see Figure 6.2). Smallpox is a serious and contagious infectious disease, and, for centuries, populations were decimated by its repeated outbreaks. Historically, the disease killed as many as 30 percent of those who became infected, and it was responsible for the deaths of such historical figures as Queen Mary II of England, Emperor Joseph I of Austria, King Luis I of Spain, Tsar Peter II of Russia, Queen Ulrika Elenora of Sweden, and King Louis XV of France. Even if death did not occur as a result of the infection, about 65–80 percent of the survivors were scarred with deep pockmarks, most prominently on the face, causing ongoing anguish even after the active disease had passed.

Two clinical varieties of smallpox are described: variola major and variola minor. Variola major is the most common form and is characterized by an

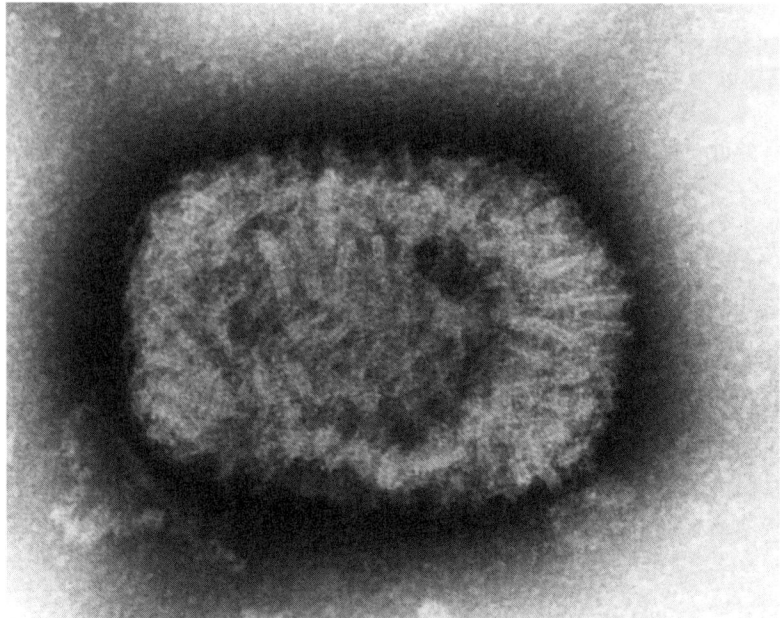

Figure 6.2. Variola (Smallpox) Virus. A highly magnified transmission electron micrograph of a single variola virion, the cause of smallpox. Image used with permission, courtesy of the CDC.

extensive rash and high fever (thus the basis for the name, derived from the Latin word for "spotted"). Variola major is further divided into four subtypes:

- ordinary: the most frequent type of smallpox, accounting for as many as 90 percent or more of cases
- modified: a mild form of smallpox that occurs in people who have previously been vaccinated (see Figure 6.3)
- flat: a severe form of smallpox with a high mortality rate
- hemorrhagic: a rare form of smallpox that is very severe and very deadly

Whereas the overall mortality rate of variola major smallpox is estimated to be 30 percent, variola minor is a less common and much less severe presentation of smallpox, with death rates of 1 percent or less. There is not a cure for smallpox, but, amazingly, a successful vaccination campaign has completely negated the influence of smallpox as a disease process affecting humankind. As of 1949, smallpox was considered eradicated from the United States, and,

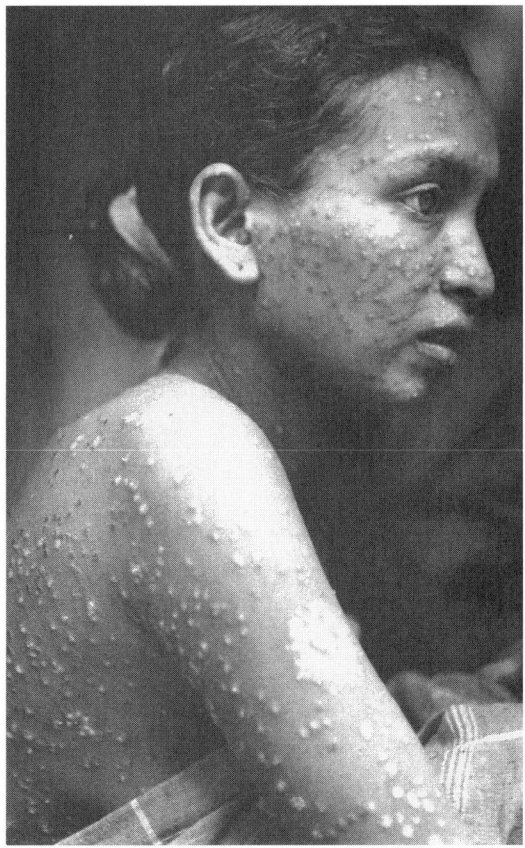

Figure 6.3. Modified Smallpox. Example of the smallpox rash seen in the modified form of the disease. Image credited to Cynthia Goldsmith; used with permission, courtesy of the CDC.

with WHO promoting a global vaccination program, smallpox was officially eradicated worldwide in 1977.

As early as 1000 B.C., a process known as "variolation" was described. This referred to a technique in which pus or scabs taken from active smallpox lesions on one patient were rubbed into the skin of another. Although the technique was not always successful in preventing smallpox infection, it did reduce the death rate among people already infected. Variolation was not immediately in favor with the general population, but the process spread with increasingly frequency across Europe and to America after the princess of Wales chose to have her own children variolated in 1717.

Edward Jenner (1749–1823), a physician in Glouchestershire, England, was intrigued by the success of variolation. He also noticed that milkmaids who had been infected with cowpox did not seem to become infected with smallpox. Cowpox, despite being caused by a virus related to smallpox, did not cause either the scarring symptoms or the high risk of death seen in smallpox. Hypothesizing that the idea behind the process of variolation might work with cowpox, Jenner bravely performed his experiment: he injected cowpox into a healthy young boy and then exposed the boy to smallpox. The boy did not develop any smallpox lesions, and Jenner called the process vaccination (taken from the Latin term *vacca*, meaning cow). Although the medical community did not accept vaccination as a legitimate technique for some time, eventually it won favor and many citizens of England and America (and ultimately, the world) were vaccinated, leading to eradication of the disease known as smallpox.

Although Jenner was brilliant enough to establish his technique based on pure clinical observation and experimentation, advances in medical science and technology have since allowed a greater understanding of vaccination. The concept of vaccination is fairly simple, actually. In response to exposure to an infectious agent, the human body produces proteins called antibodies, which neutralize or destroy the infectious agent, hopefully stopping the disease process. Antibodies are disease specific, meaning that influenza antibodies produced in response to infection with the influenza virus will only work against the flu. Thus, by administering low levels of an infectious agent, or an agent so similar that it "tricks" the body, in the form of a vaccine, antibodies can be produced for future protection against the disease. This protected state is known as immunity.

While the general concept behind vaccination is easily understood, the issues that surround successful influenza vaccination are fairly complicated. As has been discussed in previous chapters, the influenza virus is well known for its ability to mutate. The various HA and NA antigens that can be expressed by the virus from season to season have rendered a one-time, universal vaccine for influenza nonexistent to date. Instead, scientists at 110 national influenza surveillance centers and four WHO laboratories (spread across eighty-two countries) collect and analyze the data on the influenza viruses that circulate in the human population. Each year, they identify two influenza A strains and one influenza B strain that are the most likely to cause epidemics in the next season (see Figure 6.4). Vaccine manufacturers then incorporate all three strains into the vaccine composition that will be used for that year. If a chosen strain has been used previously, the process for vaccine production is faster.

Despite the difficulties in determining the composition of the annual influenza vaccine, it is clear that vaccination remains the primary method for preventing and controlling influenza. In addition to reduction in individual cases

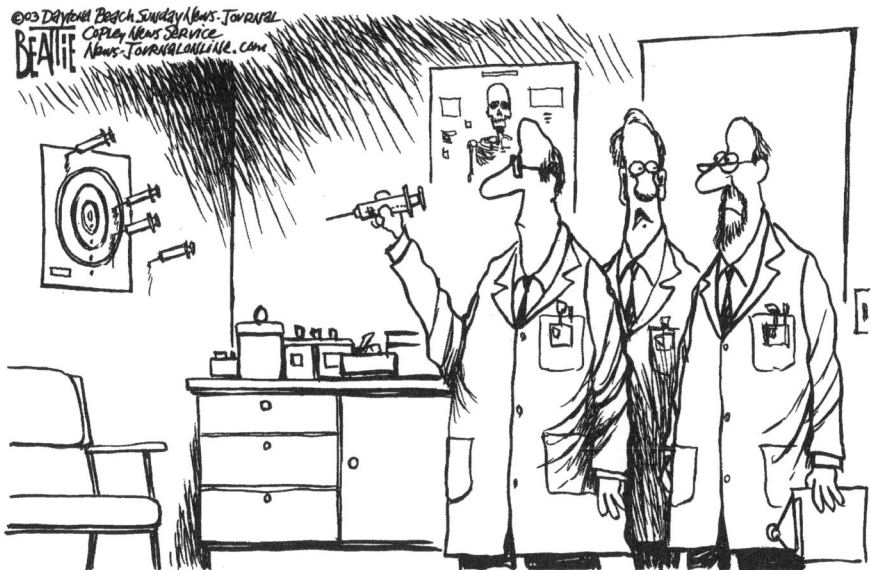

"I hate it when we're not sure we're inoculating against the right strain of flu virus."

Figure 6.4. Influenza Vaccination Cartoon. A cartoon by Beattie exemplifying the difficulties in determining the appropriate strains to include in the vaccination to attempt to thwart the following season's circulating virus. Copley News Service and Bruce Beattie.

of influenza, use of the vaccination has shown great benefit for individuals at high risk for complications of the illness. In one study of high-risk adults between the ages of eighteen and sixty-four, vaccination prevented 78 percent of deaths, 87 percent of hospitalizations, and 26 percent of general practitioner visits. In elderly patients aged sixty-five or older, 50 percent of deaths and 48 percent of hospitalizations were prevented by vaccination. Vaccination also provides indirect benefits: vaccination of children and healthcare workers, both known to spread influenza efficiently, reduces transmission of the infection to others. Vaccination can also be both cost effective and cost saving, with a substantial economic benefit attributable to such factors as reduced parental work loss days for the care of sick children, decreased work absenteeism in adults, and decreased healthcare costs, particularly in the elderly and high-risk populations.

Currently, there are several types of influenza vaccines available: killed virus vaccines and live virus vaccines.

Killed Virus Vaccines

Production of the killed virus vaccines involves multiple manufacturing steps: (1) A reference laboratory (often the CDC) grows each of the selected strains in combination with a strain called PR8. PR8 is a laboratory raised strain of infection, inactive, and unable to replicate in humans. (2) Reassortment occurs, resulting in a virus that contains six of the PR8 genes, along with the HA and NA of the seasonal strain. (3) The new reassorted virus is incubated in embryonated hens' eggs for two to three days. (4) The allantoic fluid is harvested, and the viral particles are purified at a specific density by centrifugation in a solution of increasing density. (5) The viruses are inactivated using formaldehyde or beta-propiolactone.

At this point, the vaccine production can be continued as a whole virus vaccine or a split (or subunit) virus vaccine. In a split virus vaccine, the centrifuged viral particles are washed with a detergent or ether, and the HA and NA are purified as the other viral components are removed. The split or subunit vaccines appear to cause fewer local reactions when administered compared with the whole virus vaccines, and a single dose produces an adequate antibody reaction in a population exposed to similar viruses. However, this is not believed to be sufficient if a new influenza strain emerges, and that two doses will be required for immunity in the event of a pandemic.

The remaining vaccine production steps then include the following: (6) The concentrations are standardized by the amount of hemagglutination that occurs. (7) The strains are tested to ensure adequate yield, purity, and potency. (8) The three strains (all produced separately) are combined into one vaccine. (9) The content of the combined vaccine is verified. (10) The combined vaccine is packaged into syringes for distribution. The killed virus vaccine is known as the trivalent inactivated influenza vaccine, or TIV, and is injected into the muscle of the shoulder or thigh (although other routes of administration are being investigated). It is approved for use in those age six months or older.

Side effects to the killed virus vaccine can include the following:

- GBS: rare, with an annual reporting rate of 0.04 in 2002–2003
- localized injection site reactions: pain, redness, and swelling lasting one to two days (reported in 10–64 percent of patients)
- systemic side effects: headache, fever, malaise, and myalgias (reported in 5 percent of patients)

It should be noted that the inactivated vaccines do not contain a live virus and cannot cause infection with influenza. The side effects are mostly attributable to an immune response associated with a release of interferon. Contraindications to receiving the influenza vaccine include egg allergy (because eggs are used in the inoculation procedure) and the presence of an active febrile illness.

Live Virus Vaccines

The live virus vaccine for influenza consists of a master attenuated virus into which the HA and NA genes have been inserted. The master virus is "cold adapted," which means that it replicates at an ideal temperature of twenty-five degrees Celsius. Thus, in the normal human body with a normal body temperature of thirty-seven degrees Celsius, the virus is attenuated and less likely to cause infection. The live virus vaccine is known as the live intranasal influenza vaccine, or LAIV. It is given as a nasal spray and is approved for use in healthy people who are not pregnant.

Side effects to the live virus vaccine include the following:

- asthma exacerbations: primarily reported in children
- localized symptoms: rarely, runny nose, congestion, sore throat, and headache
- systemic symptoms: abdominal pain, vomiting, and myalgias

Although side effects are rare, the live virus vaccines should not be given to immune-compromised individuals or those who may come in contact with immunocompromised patients. Other contraindications to live virus vaccination include age less than five years or older than sixty-five years, previous GBS, and children under the age of eighteen who are receiving aspirin therapy.

Currently, the world's production capacity is estimated to be about 300 million influenza vaccines per year. If the strain selection for a given year's vaccine is appropriate, it can prevent influenza in 60–90 percent of healthy adults up to age sixty-five. Unfortunately, the "best guess" approach is not always successful, as is perhaps best demonstrated by the events surrounding the swine flu vaccine produced in 1976.

In January of 1976, David Lewis, a young private at Fort Dix (a U.S. Army training center in New Jersey), began to feel ill. He felt feverish and complained of dizziness, nausea, fatigue, and muscle aches. With concern for his health and for those around him that might be at risk for becoming ill, his medical officer assigned Lewis to his quarters. Determined to perform well in his duties, Lewis instead chose to join his platoon for a planned all-night hike, which was to be done wearing a fifty-pound backpack in the bitter cold. After several hours of marching, he collapsed and was taken to the hospital. Within hours, Lewis was dead. His diagnosis? Influenza.

By the end of that same month, at least 300 recruits at Fort Dix were sick with influenza. By testing samples taken from the ill soldiers (including a specimen from Lewis' autopsy), a team of scientists at the New Jersey State Health Department Laboratory was able to determine that the Fort Dix patients had antibodies that neutralized the swine flu initially isolated by Richard Shope. As had been proven by Shope, people who were alive during the 1918 pandemic also had antibodies against his pig virus. With this connection identified, it was suggested that the Fort Dix flu strain might be the same as, or at least similar to, the influenza strain of the 1918 pandemic.

The CDC in Atlanta, Georgia, was notified, and it quickly repeated the testing and confirmed the results. With additional study, the infecting influenza strain found in the washings of some of the soldiers was identified as H1N1. Interestingly, this was notably different from the prevalent seasonal strain of flu that had already been identified in 1976, which was H3N2; this strain had also been found in some of the soldiers' specimens. So, with the confirmation of test results from the CDC, the worry for similarities to the 1918 H1N1 viral strain, and the death of a young healthy male (who was surrounded by numerous sick contacts at a military base) causing significant concern for an evolving pandemic, the government responded. On March 24th, a group of eminent scientists gathered at the White House; the group agreed that mass vaccination was indicated for a possible evolving swine flu pandemic. President Ford went on national television later that evening, saying, "I am asking the Congress to appropriate $135 million, prior to the April recess, for the production of sufficient vaccine to inoculate every man, woman, and child in the United States." Congress, as a whole, supported their president as expected, although there were several members who voiced quiet disagreement.

With the quick movement of the vaccine campaign already initiated, some members of Congress exploited the President's immunization bill by attaching $1.8 billion worth of social service spending and environmental protection funds. Adding more financial worry, the pharmaceutical manufacturers took advantage of their position and told President Ford that, because their insurance carriers would not cover them for such urgently produced vaccines, the government would have to absorb all liability for possible ill effects from the vaccine. In August, President Ford signed the National Swine Flu Immunization Program of 1976, and vaccination officially began on October 1, 1976 (see Figure 6.5).

Progress on the vaccination campaign stalled within two weeks as the report of three elderly patients' deaths was noted within days of receiving the

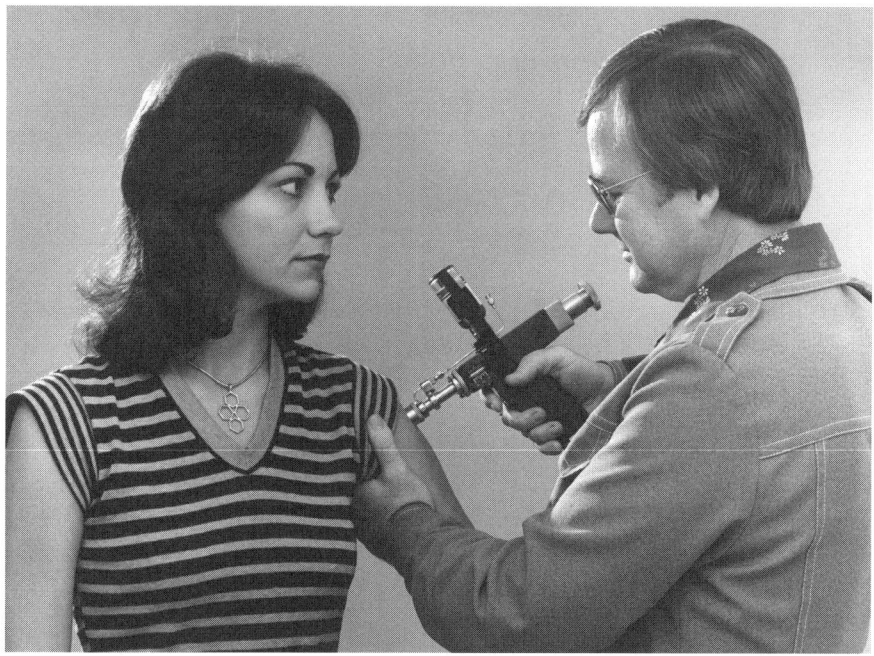

Figure 6.5. Swine Flu Vaccination. Demonstration of the administration of the swine flu vaccine in 1976. Image credited to Cynthia Goldsmith; used with permission, courtesy of the CDC.

swine flu shot. Although these deaths eventually were concluded to be incidental, and not in any way related to the vaccination, the public perception had already been influenced. Then, in November of 1976, a man in Minnesota noticed increasing weakness of his arms and legs, just days after getting the vaccination. Eventually, the man had full loss of reflexes and loss of all feeling in his hands and feet; essentially, he became paralyzed. His physician diagnosed the condition GBS and reported the event to the CDC. This first case report was quickly followed by documentation of others, and, ultimately, more than 1,100 cases of GBS were reported, about half of which were in individuals who received the vaccination. Fifty-eight people died with the diagnosis of GBS. This prompted an ensuing legal nightmare, with 4,181 claims filed with the U.S. Attorney General's office on behalf of clients alleging they had suffered ailments of various kinds as a result of the swine flu vaccine; these claims totaled $3.2 billion. Over the next fifteen years, the U.S. government would settle 393 claims for $37,789,000. Another 1,605 cases would end up in the courtroom, with fifty-three ending in judgments against the U.S. government (costing $17 million); fifty-six were lost in litigation, costing $30,683,000.

The Swine Flu Immunization Program of 1976 was a financial and political disaster. President Ford lost his reelection bid and was defeated in November of 1976 by Jimmy Carter. Ironically, influenza remained relatively rare overall in 1976, even among people who had not received the vaccine. No other deaths occurred at Fort Dix, and most of the infections that year were attributable to the H3N2 strain, sometimes in combination with a bacterial infection due to Pfeiffer's bacillus.

Chemoprophylaxis

It has been shown that, when properly used, prophylactic antiviral treatment can be quite effective in preventing infection with influenza. Dosing should be started in anticipation of an influenza A outbreak and before or after contact with individuals with documented or highly suspected influenza A illness. Unfortunately, as mentioned earlier in this chapter, resistance issues with the M2 inhibitors have resulted in a CDC-directed recommendation to avoid amantadine and rimantadine for the 2007–2008 influenza season as either treatment alternatives or for chemoprophylaxis; however, review of the original dosing instructions for the M2 inhibitors is described below. The neuraminidase inhibitors are still recommended for chemoprophylaxis: oseltamivir is approved for prevention of influenza in patients one year or older, and zanamivir is approved for prevention of influenza in persons five years and older.

M2 Inhibitors

Daily prophylaxis with an M2 inhibitor during the influenza season reduces infection rates by 50–90 percent. Postexposure prophylaxis may not be as protective.

- Amantadine should be continued daily for at least ten days after a known exposure. If amantadine is used in conjunction with the killed virus vaccine until protective antibody responses develop, then it should be administered for two to four weeks after the vaccine has been given. When the vaccine is unavailable or contraindicated, amantadine should be administered for the duration of known influenza A outbreak in the community because of repeated and unknown exposure.
- For adults and adolescents (aged ten years or older), the recommended dose of rimantadine for prevention of influenza is 100 mg twice a day. In patients with severe liver dysfunction or kidney failure and in elderly nursing home patients, a dose reduction to 100 mg daily is recommended. In children less than ten years of age, rimantadine should be administered once a day, at a dose of 5 mg/kg, but not exceeding 150 mg.

Neuraminidase Inhibitors

When given at the start of an influenza outbreak, the neuraminidase inhibitors reduce the risk of developing influenza by 60–90 percent.

- The recommended oral dose of oseltamivir for prophylaxis of influenza in adults and adolescents thirteen years and older after close contact with an infected individual is 75 mg once daily for at least ten days. Therapy should begin within two days of exposure. For pediatric patients one year and older, the dose is 2.5 mL (one half a teaspoon) for children weighing 15 kg or less, 3.8 mL (three quarters teaspoon) for children weighing 16–23 kg, 5.0 mL (one teaspoon) for children weighing 24–40 kg, and 6.2 mL (one and one quarter teaspoon) for children weighing more than 40 kg, for ten days. Dose adjustment is recommended for patients with kidney failure; in these patients, the dose should be reduced to 75 mg every other day or 30 mg every day.
- For prevention of influenza using zanamivir, the adult and adolescent dosage recommendation is two oral inhalations at 5 mg per inhalation once daily for ten to fourteen days until a vaccine response takes place or for the remainder of the exposure.

AREAS OF FUTURE RESEARCH FOR TREATMENT AND PREVENTION OF INFLUENZA

With H5N1 strains of influenza now having been identified in humans, treatment alternatives have been proposed. Oseltamivir is considered the drug of choice, with recommendations to increase the dose to 150 mg twice a day in adults with severe disease for a longer duration (at least seven to ten days or longer). It is thought that treatment with oseltamivir may still be warranted up to eight days after the onset of symptoms, if there is evidence of ongoing viral replication. Investigational antiviral agents to target influenza include novel NA inhibitors, long-acting topical NA inhibitors, conjugated sialidase, HA inhibitors, small interfering RNA, polymerase inhibitors, and protease inhibitors. Some discussion of the benefit of corticosteroids in the setting of influenza infection also exists, but results in clinical situations have been variable.

Vaccination against influenza remains the best weapon available to fight the seasonal illness that has plagued humankind for centuries. Today's concern, however, is whether vaccination in the face of a pandemic will offer any benefit to the victims. Initial approaches to the development of a vaccination targeting avian influenza have dealt with the H5N1 strain in several ways: (1) using a related but not highly pathogenic H5 virus, (2) using recombinant techniques to express the HA without involving live virus, and (3) using reverse genetic manipulation of the HA to remove the sequence responsible for high cleavability. Initial study response to use of the H5 virus was poor. Studies involving the recombinant HA technique demonstrated a dose-response relationship, indicating that the vaccine would provide benefit only at the highest doses. A more recent study of 451 adults randomly assigned subjects to receive two doses of an H5N1 vaccine of 90, 45, 15, or 7.5 micrograms of HA antigen or placebo, and they were followed for fifty-six days. A greater frequency of antibody response was seen in the subjects that received the higher dosages of HA, and the majority of subjects (58 percent) receiving the 90 µg dose had enough of an antibody response to suggest that they would be protected against the virus; however, use of the high dose is considered to be impractical in real clinical situations. Other investigational approaches include nasal inactivated vaccines, vaccines that provide cross-protective peptides or epitopes, virus-like particles, live vaccines other than cold-adapted influenza vaccine, vectored vaccines, and DNA vaccines.

In addition to the concern of producing a vaccine that will have benefit against the desired strain of influenza A, another issue is how to produce such vaccines more quickly. When a pandemic occurs, pharmaceutical companies must manufacture a vaccine as quickly as possible, while making sure the vaccine is both safe and effective. The time to produce, test, and distribute a new flu vaccine ranges between seven and eight months, so it is virtually impossible to produce an adequate amount of vaccine during a pandemic. In the United States, the national vaccine strategy is to stockpile 20 million courses of pre-pandemic vaccine and to accelerate vaccine production capacity to produce 300 million doses of an intra-pandemic vaccine within a reasonable time period (four to six months). In addition, the current study results involving the H5N1 vaccine suggest that several dosages may need to be administered for full desired effect. A number of strategies are being investigated to improve the immunogenicity of the vaccine and allow the use of lower doses; such methods might include a booster vaccine administered along with annual vaccination schedules to prime the population, use of adjuvants to lower the dose of virus necessary for immune response, and alternative routes of administration.

The ultimate goal is, of course, to someday have a universal influenza vaccine. Although the natural antibody production of humans in response to influenza does not allow cross-protection for other strains, it has been proposed that the weak immune response might be enhanced through the use of conserved antigens in a highly immunogenic form.

Conclusions

There is properly no history; only biography.

Ralph Waldo Emerson, American Poet and Essayist

As part of the *Biographies of Disease* series, this book on influenza adheres to the concept suggested above in the quotation by Emerson. Influenza's biography is completely fascinating, yet quite sobering, to consider. Despite the fact that an illness suggestive of influenza has existed for centuries, it was not until the 1930s that medical researchers, such as Richard Shope and Christopher H. Andrewes, were able to identify its viral cause. In spite of considerable medical advancements since that time, influenza continues to affect thousands of humans annually, and men, women, and children still die of flu-related complications each year. A curative treatment is not yet available, and prevention with annual vaccination remains based, to a large extent, on an educated guess. Perhaps most concerning of all is the fact that the virus has been responsible for some of the most devastating pandemics in history and is liable to cause another such event in the near future.

As a virus, influenza is simple with regard to its structure but entirely successful in achieving its goal: replication. Consisting of an inner genome, surrounded by an envelope covered in glycoprotein spikes, the influenza virus is not considered to be a living organism. However, it can easily infect a host, use the victim's own cell machinery to synthesize its proteins, and, with impressive rapidity, make new viral particles. In triggering the immune system and subsequently making its host ill, the new virions are expelled in air droplets with a cough or a sneeze. Usually, the new influenza viruses find other unsuspecting hosts to infect, and the process begins once again.

It is actually the simplicity of the influenza virus that allows its perpetual existence. The viral genome, which encodes for only eight proteins, is composed of an RNA backbone, held together with ribose sugars and phosphates. Lacking a proofreader, RNA viruses are subject to considerable mutation. In the case of influenza, the mutations are enough to cause antigenic drift, a seasonal variation in the HA and NA glycoprotein spikes projecting from the surface of the viral particles. This not only limits the ability to accurately determine what viral strains will predominate each season but also minimizes the chance that the human antibodies produced during previous infection will allow full protection against invasion of the virus in the future. Thus, humans (and other animals) are subject to annual, seasonal attacks of influenza and have suffered from disease outbreaks at least since the time of Hippocrates.

Even more worrisome, however, is the ability of influenza to undergo antigenic shift, a reassortment of viral components from both human and avian sources, allowing production of an entirely new strain of influenza that might have the unrecognizable HA or NA components from the bird genome with the transmission tendencies of the human virus. Thus, a novel influenza strain can spread unchecked, with absolutely no historical immunity to stand in its way. It is this phenomenon that likely led to most of the previous pandemics of the twentieth century. The exception to this is the 1918 pandemic, which may have been caused by a purely avian strain of influenza that adapted to humans. Amazingly, medical researchers have been able to evacuate, isolate, and identify the influenza strain of 1918 from preserved autopsy specimens and from tissue obtained from victims buried in Alaska's permafrost. Now known as H1N1, the strain has been shown to have considerable lethality because of various factors such as enhanced replication capacity, high affinity for human respiratory epithelial cells, and mediation of the human immune response.

In most seasonal outbreaks of influenza, the great majority of cases tend to be uncomplicated. Occasionally, more severe manifestations of primary viral pneumonia or secondary bacterial pneumonia occur. More rarely still, extrapulmonary manifestations are identified. Most healthcare providers are able to identify patients with influenza by conducting a health history and physical examination. In addition, laboratory testing with rapid antigen tests, serology, or viral culture can confirm the suspected diagnosis of influenza.

Once identified, patients with influenza can be offered supportive care or, possibly, antiviral treatment (if symptoms have been present less than forty-eight hours at the time of diagnosis). Prevention of influenza is accomplished with both selective use of antiviral medications and vigilant seasonal immunization.

Currently, much attention is focused on the novel subtypes of influenza A that have more recently been identified, particularly H5N1. This avian influenza strain, initially identified in a human outbreak in Hong Kong in 1997, remains in circulation today. Although it has not yet shown impressive human-to-human transmission, it continues to mutate, to cause isolated outbreaks, and to maintain an impressive lethality for its victims. It is just such an influenza strain that causes worry for a future, potentially devastating pandemic. If mutations or reassortment of H5N1 allow more ready spread between human hosts, an outbreak could rapidly spread across the globe among a current population without any hope of an antibody response. It is not difficult to imagine the consequences: high attack rates, severe morbidity and mortality, overwhelmed medical services, shortages of healthcare providers, political nightmares, and disruption of already fragile economies. Thus, aggressive monitoring of avian influenza strains continues through the efforts of WHO, along with more than fifty countries and various international partners. Pandemic preparation is well underway, as are ongoing vaccine research and production. With such preemptive surveillance and proactive pandemic preparation, it is hoped that an event reminiscent of the 1918 outbreak can be averted or at least minimized.

The biography of influenza is rich with historical documentation, scientific discoveries, heroic adventures, unfortunate fatalities, and untiring research. Despite this attempt to convey its story in full, it is not likely to end here. Influenza's biography will continue to evolve along with humankind, and the manner in which the virus and humans will exist together remains to be seen.

Timeline

412 B.C.	Hippocrates, known as the Father of Medicine, describes an outbreak of a clinical syndrome suggestive of influenza.
212 B.C.	The Roman army is "visited by pestilence, a calamity almost heavy enough to turn them from all thoughts of war." The historian Titus Livius, known as Livy, later authors a monumental *History of Rome* and describes this outbreak, thought possibly to be attributable to influenza.
855	A virulent epidemic resembling influenza starts in Central Asia and spreads across Persia, killing a large number of people.
876	Charlemagne's conquest of Europe is slowed by a flu epidemic that spreads across the continent and claims the lives of much of his army.
1510	Possibly originating in Africa, a large outbreak of influenza rages across Europe. Although the death rate during this outbreak is low, the attack rate is high.
1557	A large outbreak of influenza is documented.

1580	The first definite and documented influenza pandemic originates in Asia during the summer months, spreads to Africa, then travels through Europe along two corridors from Asia Minor and Northwest Africa, and eventually lands in America. In some places, two waves of illness are documented, and some cities are "nearly entirely depopulated by the disease."
1688	Outbreaks of influenza are described in England, Ireland, and America, and "the people dyed … as in a plague."
1693	Additional outbreaks of influenza are documented in England, Ireland, and America. After this outbreak, it was noted that "all conditions of persons were attacked … those who were very strong and hardy were taken in the same manner as the weak and spoiled … the youngest as well as the oldest."
1699	Again, outbreaks of influenza are seen in England, Ireland, and America. Cotton Mather, a Puritan minister and author of the time, wrote in January of 1699 in Massachusetts, "The sickness extended to allmost all families. Few or none escaped, and many dyed especially in Boston, and some dyed in a strange or unusual manner, in some families all weer sick together, in some town allmost all weer sick so that it was a time of disease."
1729–1730	A pandemic of influenza, originating in Russia, travels across Europe with deaths most numerous among the elderly and pregnant women. A high attack rate and appreciable mortality overall is noted. Afterward, it was noted that, in London in particular, barely 1 percent escaped the disease.
1732–1733	An influenza epidemic of very severe and very widespread illness is documented. The site of origin is unclear but is postulated to be either Connecticut or Moscow in the fall of 1732. Eventually, the illness is found worldwide.
1742–1743	A widespread outbreak of influenza is documented in Europe.
1761–1762	An outbreak of influenza is identified in North America and the West Indies in 1761 and is followed by disease in Europe the next year.
1767	Influenza is reported in North America and most of Europe but escapes Britain.

1775–1776	Influenza is found in all of Europe and both the Near and Far East. Mortality in England is low.
1781–1782	Another influenza pandemic occurs. It is thought to have originated in China in the autumn and eventually is reported to have caused illness in all European countries, the West Indies, and North America. It afflicts two thirds of the population of Rome, followed by three quarters of the people of Britain throughout the summer of 1782.
1788–1789	An epidemic hits New England, New York, and Nova Scotia in the fall and is eventually seen throughout Europe. Most early deaths appear to be caused by infection with a secondary pneumonia, although in Britain, the disease is mild and rarely associated with death.
1800–1802	A mild disease outbreak of influenza is seen in all of Europe, China, and Brazil. The site of origin is again unclear but is postulated to be either China in September or Russia in October.
1830–1833	A pandemic begins in the winter in China, and then spreads via the sea southward to reach the Philippines, India, and Indonesia, and across Russia into Europe. It reaches North America in 1831–1832, and then recurs in Europe in 1831–1832, and again in 1832–1833.
1836–1837	Influenza occurs in Europe, parts of Africa, and Australia. The mortality rate is high in London.
1847–1848	With the exact source unclear (perhaps in Russia in March), influenza travels through Europe, North America, the West Indies, and Brazil. Considerable mortality is appreciated, and, in Britain, it is referred to as "the great influenza of 1847." More people die from this pandemic than during the great cholera epidemic of 1832.
1850–1851	Influenza is seen in North and South America, the West Indies, Australia, and Germany.
1857–1858	A widespread outbreak of influenza originates in Panama in August and spreads through North and South America, as well as Europe. Many deaths occur in Rome, and it is referred to as "one of the greatest epidemics."

1873–1875	Influenza is identified in North America and the European Continent. Britain is spared the outbreak.
1876	Robert Koch isolates and identifies the anthrax bacteria, confirming the validity of the germ theory of disease.
1884	Koch's postulates are published in a medical journal entitled *The Etiology of Tuberculosis.*
1889–1890	A worldwide influenza epidemic begins in Central Asia, spreads north into Russia, east to China, and west to Europe. It eventually strikes North America, parts of Africa, and the major Pacific Rim countries. Although the first wave of infection is mild with low mortality rates, the subsequent three waves of infection are severe. At least 250,000 die in Europe, and, worldwide, the deaths total 500,000–750,000. The epidemic is thereafter known as "the Russian Flu." The strain is ultimately identified as H2N2.
1892	Dmitri Ivanovski publishes evidence of an infectious agent found after using a filter that retains bacteria, suggesting that viruses may cause disease. Also in this year, Richard Pfeiffer identifies a bacillus and states that it is the cause of influenza.
1899	Martinus Beijerinck recognizes "soluble" living microbes and essentially allows the concept and terminology of a virus to be described.
1900	A major influenza epidemic occurs in North American, England, and Wales. The strain is identified as H3N2.
1918–1920	"The Spanish Flu" pandemic occurs. It is the most lethal outbreak ever and kills an estimated 50 million people worldwide. Three separate waves of illness occur in less than twelve months. The first wave in the spring of 1918 is mild, but the second wave in the autumn of 1918 is severe. Half of the deaths are in young adults aged twenty to forty. A third wave begins early in 1919, with continued mortality in young adults. The strain is identified as H1N1.
1930	Richard Shope confirms that swine influenza is caused by a virus and suspects it may be a similar causative agent that results in human influenza.

1933	Sir Christopher Andrewes, Wilson Smith, and Sir Patrick Laidlaw confirm that influenza in humans is caused by a virus. Shope determines that it is similar to swine influenza virus but not identical.
1940	Frank Macfarlane Burnet "grows" influenza on a laboratory system comprised embryonated chicken eggs. Thomas Francis isolates the influenza B virus.
1941	It is discovered that influenza causes hemagglutination of red blood cells, providing a new assay for the virus.
1946	An influenza variant is detected in Australia and eventually spreads worldwide. It does not give rise to a major epidemic.
1949	R. M. Taylor isolates the influenza C virus.
1957–1958	"The Asian Flu" starts in China in February and spreads through the Pacific, eventually reaching Europe and the United States in June. A second wave follows. The strain is identified as H2N2.
1968–1969	"The Hong Kong Flu" originates in southeast China in July and eventually kills thousands of people worldwide. However, the characteristics of the outbreak vary, with 80,000 deaths in the United States in the first wave but low initial mortality in Europe. In the second wave, considerable mortality is demonstrated in Europe, with an estimated 30,000 deaths in an eight-week period in Britain alone. The strain is identified as H3N2, a virus still in circulation today.
1976	The swine flu is found in a young army recruit at Fort Dix in New Jersey, prompting a new pandemic fear. This leads to a massive influenza immunization program at the order of the president. The vaccinations become associated with Guillian-Barré syndrome, an ascending paralysis, which kills 5 percent of those afflicted.
1977	Appearance of a new strain in humans called "the Russian Flu" is identified as H1N1. Isolated in northern China, it is similar to the virus seen before 1957. The outbreak affects primarily young individuals who were born after the previous H1N1 viruses had last circulated (i.e., after 1957).

1986	An Avian variation of swine flu in the Netherlands is identified.
1988	Swine flu kills a pregnant woman.
1993	A strain of swine flu in the Netherlands sickens two children.
1995	One adult contracts conjunctivitis in the United Kingdom after infection with a duck influenza virus.
1997	The "Hong Kong Poultry Virus" infects at least eighteen people, killing six of them. The strain is identified as H5N1. This documents the first time an influenza virus has been transmitted directly from birds to humans. Public health authorities mandate that every single chicken in Hong Kong must be slaughtered; 1.2 million birds are killed. A vaccine is developed.
1999	A strain identified as H9N2 appears for the first time in humans, causing illness in two children in Hong Kong. Poultry is the probable source.
2002	Identified as H7N2, a new strain appears in one person in Virginia after an outbreak in poultry.
2003	A strain identified as H5N1 causes illness in two Hong Kong family members after a visit to China; one of them dies. Another family member dies of an undiagnosed respiratory illness. This is the same strain that caused the outbreak in 1997 in Hong Kong; the strain continues to survive in chickens.

A strain identified as H7N7 is found in poultry farms in the Netherlands, Belgium, and Germany. All victims become ill with eye infections or flu-like illness; most are poultry workers. A veterinarian who visited an affected poultry farm dies. Pigs are also infected. Public health authorities kill nearly 30 million poultry and swine.

A strain identified as H7N2 causes hospitalization of a patient in New York.

A strain identified as H9N2 causes illness in one child in Hong Kong. |
| **2004** | An H5N1 strain causes illness in forty-seven people in Thailand and Vietnam; thirty-four die.

A strain identified as H7N3 is reported for the first time in humans with illness in two poultry workers in Canada. |

A strain identified as H10N7 is reported for the first time in humans with illness in two infants in Egypt. One child's father is a poultry worker.

2005   A strain identified as H5N1 is found in a human case in Cambodia in February. By May, four cases are reported, and all are fatal. A case in Indonesia occurs in July, also fatal. Seven cases of laboratory-confirmed illness over the next three months are identified in Indonesia; four are fatal. By December 30th, 142 laboratory-confirmed cases are described in Asia, with seventy-four deaths.

2006   A strain identified as H5N1 causes two fatal cases in Turkey. In January, China reports ten cases with seven deaths. Iraq reports a fatal case. In March, seven cases with five deaths in Azerbaijan are reported. In April, four cases with two deaths in Egypt are identified, and, in May, a case in Africa is noted.

2007   A strain identified as H5N1 causes deaths in Africa and Lao People's Democratic Republic. Vietnam reports its first human cases since 2005 in two isolated young males from Vinh Phuc and Thai Nguyen. Myanmar confirms its first human case in a seven year old from Shan State. Eight people test positive in the North West Frontier Province of Pakistan.

An avian influenza strain identified as H9N2 is found in a nine-month-old female from China; the illness is mild.

A resolution to provide international sharing of influenza viruses is reached at the World Health Organization World Health Assembly in Geneva.

The United Kingdom Health Protection reports at least four human infections with a low pathogenic avian influenza strain, identified as H7N2. The cases are associated with concurrent poultry infection.

Glossary

Adult respiratory distress syndrome (ARDS): Progression of pulmonary damage that can be triggered by influenza infection, leading to increased morbidity and mortality.

Antibody: A molecule produced by plasma cells that can bind to an infectious agent at an antigenic site as a means of defense offered by the immune system of the host.

Antigen: Any substance, including viral particles, that induces a specific host immune response and provides a means of reacting with immune-mediated molecules, such as antibodies.

Antigenic drift: Progressive accumulation of mutations in the influenza virus acquired over time. This phenomenon results in ongoing seasonal influenza outbreaks and the need to modify the influenza vaccine each year.

Antigenic shift: Recombination of zoonotic influenza strains with human strains, resulting in drastic alteration in the viral HA and NA structures. This phenomenon leads to a previously unrecognized influenza strain, which can potentially lead to a devastating pandemic.

Arthralgia: Pain present in a joint.

Asian Flu: Refers to the influenza strain H2N2, which caused the documented pandemic in 1957.

Avian influenza: Influenza caused by a strain of virus known to exist in the avian population.

Bacteria: A unicellular but living organism that can cause a variety of infectious diseases.

Bacteriophage: A virus that can infect bacteria, with incorporation of the viral genetic material into the intimate workings of the cell.

Bleeding: A primitive treatment modality using release of blood from a vessel for purported therapeutic benefit.

Cellular immunity: The white blood cell response to immune system activation, which allows the targeting and destruction of host cells infected with a foreign invader.

Centrifugation: A process of separation of lighter portions of a mixture from the heavier portions by centrifugal (moving away from a center) force.

Cephalgia: Ache in the head.

Chemoprophylaxis: Use of an antiviral medication to prevent the development of the influenza disease process.

Croup: A condition characterized by a barking cough, hoarseness, and stridor, usually occurring as a result of infection with a respiratory virus such as influenza.

Cupping: A primitive treatment modality using a flame to absorb oxygen and create a vacuum in a glass container, which was then placed on the body. In dry cupping, the glass was placed on intact skin to stimulate blood flow; in wet cupping, the glass was placed over incised skin to help facilitate removal of blood.

Cyanosis: A bluish discoloration of the tissue caused by poor oxygenation, most pronounced at the skin and mucous membranes.

Deoxyribonucleic acid (DNA): A strand of genetic material composed of deoxyribose sugars and phosphates to complement a backbone of four base chemicals, including cytosine, guanine, adenine, and thymine.

Differential diagnosis: A list of possible diagnoses that could be considered as cause of a patient's disease, based on systematic comparison of clinical findings.

Encephalitis: Inflammation of the brain, often leading to confusion, which can occur as a complication of infection with influenza.

Epidemic: An outbreak of influenza that is confined to one location, such as city or country, occurring suddenly in numbers in excess of normal seasonal expectations.

Fever: Elevation of the body temperature above normal.

Fungi: Mold or yeast forms that exist in the microbiological domain of *Eukaryota*.

Genome: The complete genetic code found within an organism.

Glycoprotein: Protein projections or spikes protruding from the influenza viral envelope, consisting of either hemagglutinin or neuraminidase.

Guillan-Barré Syndrome (GBS): An autoimmune disorder characterized by ascending paralysis, described in association with influenza infection and vaccination.

Hemadsorption: The adherence of red blood cells to other surfaces, such as other cells or particles.

Hemagglutinin (HA): A glycoprotein antigenic site projecting from the influenza viral envelope, which allows attachment of the virus to the cell of a host.

Hong Kong Flu: The influenza strain H3N2, which caused the pandemic of 1968.

Humoral immunity: Production of antibodies by the host immune system in response to infection by a foreign invader.

Incubation period: The duration of time between acquisition of the influenza virus to the onset of identifiable symptoms of disease.

Koch's postulates: A set of criteria designed to aid in establishing a link between an infectious agent and a resulting disease process.

Miasma: A "foulness" in the air, possibly emanating originally from the soil or earth, that was thought to cause disease.

Morbidity: The incidence or prevalence of a disease state.

Mortality: The incidence or prevalence of death from a disease state.

Myalgia: Pain in a muscle or muscle group.

Myocarditis: Inflammation of the walls of the heart muscle.

Myositis: Inflammation of a voluntary muscle.

Neuraminidase (NA): A glycoprotein antigen site projecting from the influenza viral envelope, which allows full penetration of the virus into a host cell and separation from the host cell after replication.

*Orthomyxoviridae***:** A family of RNA viruses, including influenza viruses A, B, and C.

Outbreak: Seasonal bouts of influenza infection in a population.

Pandemic: Evolution of an epidemic with spread throughout the world, caused by a new influenza viral strain not seen previously in human circulation.

Parasites: Simple infectious agents of a diverse nature that live on or within another organism and can cause a variety of diseases in the host.

Pathogen: An infectious agent capable of producing disease in its host.

Pathogenicity: The quality or ability of an infectious agent to cause disease in its host or target.

Pericarditis: Inflammation of the sac that surrounds the heart.

Pfeiffer's bacillus (*Bacillus influenzae***):** A bacterium identified by Richard Friedrich Johannes Pfeiffer, thought at one time to be the cause of influenza. The bacterium is now known as *Haemophilus influenzae*.

Placebo: A "dummy" medical treatment used as a control in a clinical trial or as a therapy given solely for psychosomatic benefit.

Plasmapheresis: Removal of plasma from a sick patient, followed by replacement with formed elements of the donor plasma and other transfusion substances.

Polymerase chain reaction (PCR): An amplification technique that allows millions of copies to be made from a single fragment of a gene.

Purulent: Pertaining to the appearance of pus, an inflammatory mixture of cells, proteins, and fluid.

Rapid antigen test: Laboratory test allowing immunological detection of influenza viral antigen in respiratory secretions.

Replication: Use of a viral genome to produce more viral particles.

Reye's syndrome: An illness manifesting in confusion and liver disease, associated with use of aspirin in younger children during a viral illness.

Ribonucleic acid (RNA): A strand of genetic material composed of four different chemicals within a backbone, held together with ribose sugars and phosphates. The four base chemicals include adenine, guanine, cytosine, and uracil.

Ribosome: A large molecule that is the site of protein synthesis in host cells.

Rigors: Involuntary shaking chills accompanied by a sense of coldness.

Sensitivity: The probability that a person suffering from a disease will also have a positive test confirming the diagnosis; a true positive.

Spanish Flu: The influenza strain H1N1, which caused the pandemic of 1918.

Specificity: The probability that a person without a disease state will also test negative for the diagnosis; a true negative.

Stridor: A harsh, high-pitched sound heard during inspiration as a result of laryngeal obstruction.

Toxic shock syndrome (TSS): A syndrome of inflammatory symptoms caused by toxin release during infection with *Staphylococcus aureus* bacteria.

Translation: Synthesis of proteins based on the genomic template.

Transverse myelitis: Inflammation of the spinal cord along a cross-section, inducing neurological symptoms.

Tumor necrosis factor: A type of cytokine toxin released during host immune system activation in response to infection.

Variola: The virus that causes smallpox.

Variolation: A technique in which pus or scabs taken from active smallpox lesions were rubbed into skin in an attempt to prevent future smallpox infection.

Virion: A single viral particle, essentially composed of genetic material surrounded by a protective layer.

Virulence: The degree to which an infectious agent can invade its host and cause disease manifestations.

Virus: An infectious agent, generally not thought to be alive, with the ability to reproduce via replication in living host cells.

Zoonotic: An animal source that can facilitate transfer of an infectious agent to man.

Bibliography

Andrewes, C. H. 1956. "Influenza: Theme and Variations." *California Medicine* 84:375–380.

Andrewes, C. H. 1973. "Fifty Years with Viruses." *Annual Review of Microbiology* 27:1–14.

Barry, J. M. 2004. *The Great Influenza: The Epic Story of the Deadliest Plague in History.* New York: Viking, The Penguin Group.

Bates, B. 1991. *A Guide to Physical Examination and History Taking,* 5th edition. Philadelphia: J. B. Lippincott Company.

Beckman, H. B., Frankel, R. M. 1984. "The Effect of Physician Behavior on the Collection of Data." *Annals of Internal Medicine* 102:520–528.

Beveridge, W. I. B. 1977. *Influenza: The Last Great Plague.* New York: Prodist, Neale Watson Academic Publications, Inc.

Black, M., Armstrong, P. 2006. *An Introduction to Avian and Pandemic Influenza,.* http://www.health.nsw.gov.au/public-health/phb/HTML2006/julaug06html/article2p99.html.

Blaser, M. J. 2006. "Pandemics and Preparations." *Journal of Infectious Diseases* 194: S70–S72.

Bureau of Public Affairs Fact Sheet. 2007. *U.S. Government Support to Combat Avian and Pandemic Influenza—An Update,* http://www.state.gov/r/pa/scp/86190.htm.

Cather, W. 2007. *One of Ours.* Mineola, MN: Dover Publications, Inc.

Crosby, A. W. 2003. *America's Forgotten Pandemic: The Influenza of 1918*, 2nd edition. New York: Cambridge University Press.

Davies, P. 2000. *The Devil's Flu: The World's Deadliest Influenza Epidemic and the Scientific Hunt for the Virus that Caused It.* New York: Henry Holt and Company, LLC.

Ebell, M. H., White, L. L., Casault, T. 2004. "A Systematic Review of the History and Physical Examination to Diagnose Influenza." *Journal of the American Board of Family Physicians* 17:1–5.

Fauci, A. S. 2006. "Seasonal and Pandemic Influenza Preparedness: Science and Countermeasures." *Journal of Infectious Diseases* 194:S73–S76.

Fernandez, Elizabeth. 2002. *The Virus Detective: Dr. John Hultin Has Found Evidence of the 1918 Flu Epidemic That Has Eluded Experts for Decades*, http://www.sfgate.com/cgi-bin/article.cgi?file=/chronicle/archive/2002/02/17/CM40502.DTL.

Fiore, A. E., Shay, D. K., Haber, P., Iskander, J.K., Uyeki, T.M., Mootrey, G., Bresee, J.S., Cox, N.J. 2007. "Prevention and Control of Influenza: Recommendations of the Advisory Committee on Immunization Practices (ACIP), 2007." *MMWR Recommendations and Reports* 56:1–54.

García-Sastre, A., Whitley, R. J. 2006. "Lessons Learned from Reconstructing the 1918 Influenza Pandemic." *Journal of Infectious Diseases* 194:S127–S132.

Garrett, L. 1994. *The Coming Plague: Newly Emerging Disease in a World Out of Balance.* New York: Farrar, Straus and Giroux.

Hayden, F. G., Pavia, A. T. 2006. "Antiviral Management of Seasonal and Pandemic Influenza." *Journal of Infectious Diseases* 194:S119–126.

Hays, J. N. 1998. *The Burdens of Disease: Epidemics and Human Response in Western History.* New Brunswick, NJ: Rutgers University Press.

Kamps, B. S., Hoffmann, C., Preiser, W., eds. 2006. *Influenza Report*, http://www.influenzareport.com.

Karlen, A. 1995. *Man and Microbes: Disease and Plagues in History and Modern Times.* New York: G.P. Putnam's Sons.

Kolata, G. 1999. *Flu: The Story of the Great Influenza Pandemic of 1918 and the Search for the Virus That Caused It.* New York: Simon & Schuster.

Korsch, B. M., Harding, C. 1997. *The Intelligent Patient's Guide to the Doctor-Patient Relationship: Learning How to Talk so Your Doctor Will Listen.* New York: Oxford University Press.

Lehrer, Jim. 1997. *Revisiting the 1918 Flu*, http://www.pbs.org/newshour/bb/health/march97/1918_3-24.html.

McConnell, C. P. 2000. "The Treatment of Influenza." *The Journal of the American Osteopathic Association* 100:311–313.

McDonald, J. 2003. *In the Shelter of Monadnock: Jaffrey, New Hampshire, Cather's Favorite Retreat and Final Resting Place*, http://www.cather.unl.edu/community/tours/jaffrey.html.

Morens, D. M., Taubenberger, J. K. 2006. "Influenza and the Origins of the Phillips Collection, Washington, DC. *Emerging Infections Diseases* 12:78–80.

Morgan, A. 2006. "Avian Influenza: An Agricultural Perspective." *Journal of Infectious Diseases* 194:S139–S146.

Morse, S. S., ed. 1993. *Emerging Viruses*. Oxford: Oxford University Press.

National Institute of Allergy and Infectious Diseases. 2007. *Flu (Influenza): Timeline of Human Flu Pandemics*, http://www3.niaid.nih.gov/healthscience/healthtopics/Flu/Research/ongoingResearch/Pandemic/TimelineHumanPandemics.html.

New York Times. 1918. *F. D. Roosevelt Spanish Grip Victim*, http://query.nytimes.com/mem/archive-free/pdf?res=9A03E1DA1531E433A25753C2A96F9C946996D6CF.

Nichol, K. L., Treanor, J. J. 2006. "Vaccines for Seasonal and Pandemic Influenza." *Journal of Infectious Diseases* 194:S111–S118.

Nicholson, K. G., Webster, R. G., Hay, A. J., eds. 1998. 1st edition. *Textbook of Influenza*. Oxford: Blackwell Science Ltd.

Petric, M., Comanor, L., Petti, C. A. 2006. "Role of the Laboratory in Diagnosis of Influenza during Seasonal Epidemics and Potential Pandemics." *Journal of Infectious Diseases* 194:S98–S110.

Porter, K. A. 1939. *Pale Horse, Pale Rider*. New York: The Modern Library, Random House.

Potter, C. W. 2001. "A History of Influenza." *Journal of Applied Microbiology* 91:572–579.

Reeves, R. 2007. *Richard Reeves Quotes*, www.brainyquote.com/quotes/authors/r/richard_reeves.html.

Schachter, N. 2005. *The Good Doctor's Guide to Colds & Flu: How to Prevent and Treat Colds, Flu, Sinusitis, Bronchitis, Strep Throat, and Pneumonia at Any Age*. New York: HarperCollins Publishers, Inc.

Southgate, M. T. 2005. "The Cover." *Journal of the American Medical Association* 294:1733.

Starr, I. 2006. "Influenza in 1918: Recollections of the Epidemic in Philadelphia." *Annals of Internal Medicine* 145:138–140.

Survivor, M. D. 2001. *Hippocratic Oath—Classical Version*, http://www.pbs.org/wgbh/nova/doctors/oath_classical.html.

Tyrrell, D. A. J. 1991. "Christopher Howard Andrewes." *Biographical Memoirs of Fellows of the Royal Society*, 37th edition. London: The Royal Society, pp. 35–68.

U.S. Department of Health & Human Services. 2006. *Pandemic Flu*, http://www.pandemicflu.gov.

Van Epps, H. L. 2006. "Influenza: Exposing the True Killer." *Journal of Experimental Medicine* 203:803.

Walsh, E. E., Cox, C., Falsey, A. R. 2002. "Clinical Features of Influenza A Virus Infection in Older Hospitalized Persons." *Journal of the American Geriatric Society* 50:1498–1503.

Waring, J. I. 1971. *A History of Medicine in South Carolina 1900–70*. South Carolina Medical Association.

Webster, R. G., Walker, E. J. 2003. *Influenza*, www.scs.carleton.ca/~soma/biosec/readings/influenza/influenza.html.

Whitley, R. J., Monto, A. S. 2006. "Prevention and Treatment of Influenza in High-Risk Groups: Children, Pregnant Women, Immunocompromised Hosts, and Nursing Home Residents." *Journal of Infectious Diseases* 194:S133–S138.

Whitley, R. J., Monto, A. S. 2006. "Seasonal and Pandemic Influenza Preparedness: A Global Threat." *Journal of Infectious Diseases* 194:S65–S69.

Wolfe, T. 1997. *Look Homeward, Angel.* New York: Scribner Classics.

World Health Organization. 2003. *Influenza: Report by The Secretariat,* http://www.who.int/gb/ebwha/pdf_files/WHA56/ea5623.pdf.

Index

adenine, 3

adenovirus, 12, 23

Adult Respiratory Distress Syndrome (ARDS), 20, 49, 67

Advisory Committee on Immunization Practices (ACIP), 69, 70, 95

AIDS, 2; HIV infection, 69, 73

amantadine, *See* antiviral medications

Andrewes, Christopher H., 5, 9–12, 107, 115; figure of, 10

anthrax, xx, 114

antibody, 18–19, 98, 108; in serological testing, 83–84

antigen, 15, 18

antigenic drift, 25–26, 108; definition of, 25

antigenic shift, 25–26, 108; definition of, 26

antiviral medications, 88–95, 104–105, 109; amantadine, 29, 89–91, 104; amantadine, side effects of, 90–91; M2 inhibitors, 29, 88–92, 104; neuraminidase inhibitors, 29, 92–95, 105; oseltamivir, 29, 92–94, 105; oseltamivir, side effects of, 94; resistance in, 89–90, 93; rimantadine, 29, 91–92, 104; rimantadine, side effects of, 92; zanamivir, 29, 94–95, 105; zanamivir, side effects of, 94–95

Aristotle, xvii, xviii

Armed Forces Institute of Pathology, 31, 52

Arouet, François-Marie: quote from, 71

Asian flu, 24

attack rate, 22, 109, 111

avian influenza, 2, 12, 26, 108, 109, 116, 117; H5N1, 20, 26, 27–30, 53, 54–55, 109, 116, 117; H5N1, clinical manifestations of, 67; H5N1, figure of, 27; H5N1, vaccination, 105–106; H7N2,

30, 116, 117; H7N3, 30, 116; H7N7,
    30, 53, 66, 116; H9N2, 30, 116, 117;
    H10N7, 30, 117; testing for, 79

Bacillus influenzae, 4, 5. *See also* Pfeiffer's
    bacillus and *Haemophilus influenzae*
bacteria, 1–2, 64; *Mycoplasma catarrhalis*,
    7; *Staphylococcus aureus*, 2, 64, 67–68;
    Streptococcus pneumoniae, 2, 50, 64
bacteriolysis, 7
bacteriophages, 2
Bacterium pneumosintes, 6
Barré, John Alexander, 65
Beijerinck, Martinus, 114
Bell Telephone Company, 44
biphasic fever curve, 61
bleeding, 41
blood generation theory, xvii, xx
British Expeditionary Force, 32
bubonic plague, 5, 7
Burnet, Sir MacFarlane, 49–50, 115
Bush, George W., 56

Camp Lewis, 5
Carter, Jimmy, 104
Cather, Willa, 59–60, 61; *One of Ours*,
    59
cellular immunity, 18–20
Centers for Disease Control and Preven-
    tion (CDC), xxii, 69, 90, 100,
    102–103, 104
Chadwick, Sir Edwin, xvii, xx
Chamberland, Charles, xvii, xxi; filter of,
    xvii, xxi, 5, 6
Charlemagne, 111
chemoprophylaxis, 104–105
chicken pox, 2
cholera, xx, 1, 5, 7
cilia, 18, 60
conjunctivitis, 30, 66, 67, 77, 116
Contagium vivum fluidum, xxi
cowpox, 98
croup, 61, 66, 68

cupping, 41
cytosine, 3
cytokines, 19–20, 27–28, 49, 68:
    interferon, 19, 27–28, 101; interleu-
    kins, 19; tumor necrosis factor, 19,
    27–28

Davis, Norman, 48
deoxyribonucleic acid (DNA), 3: proof-
    reading of, 25; replication of, 3–4
differential diagnosis, 76
Dot, Admiral, 41

elemental theory, xvii, xviii
elements, xvii, xviii
Emerson, Ralph Waldo: quote from, 107
Empedocles, xvii, xviii
encephalitis, 66, 76
epidemic, 21; definition of, 22
Eukaryota, 2

Farr, William, xvii, xx
fecal-oral transmission, 3
fermentation, xx
flu, *See* influenza
Flumadine®. *See* antiviral medications
Food and Agriculture Organization
    (FAO), 56
Ford, Gerald, 102–104
Ford Motor Company, 32
Fort Dix, 101–102, 104, 115
Fowler, W., 43
Francis, Thomas, 115
Frary, Donald P., 48
fungi, 2

Galen, xvii, xviii
Garlow, Irma Cody, 42
Gates, Frederick L., 5, 6–7
Genome Sequencing Project, 56
germ theory, xvii, xx–xxi
German Plague, 49
Goodpasture, Ernest W., 50

glycoproteins, 13; hemagglutinin (HA), 13–15, 25–26, 49, 98, 108; neuraminidase (NA), 13–15, 25–26, 49, 98, 108
Gordon, Mervyn, 10
guanine, 3
Guillain, George, 65
Guillain-Barré syndrome, 65, 100, 103, 115

Haemophilus influenzae, 6, 7, 64; figure of, 6. *See also Bacillus influenzae* and Pfeiffer, bacillus
Hagadorn, Colonel Charles, 45
health history, 71–76, 108; allergies, 73; chief complaint, 72; family history, 73; history of present illness, 72; interview techniques, 74–76; medications, 73; past medical history, 73; past surgical history, 73; patient etiquette in, 75; review of systems, 73–74; social history, 73
Hemophilus influenzae suis, 8, 9
hepatitis, 2, 3
herald wave, 23
herd immunity, 34
Hippocrates, xv–xvii, 111; clinical discoveries of, xvi; quote from, xv
Hippocratic: Corpus, xv; Oath, xv–xvii
Hong Kong flu (1968), 24, 115
hookworm, 2
House, Edward, 48
Hultin, John, 51–52, 53–54
humoral immunity, 18–19, 98
humours, xviii

ill humour theory, xvii, xviii; temperaments of: choleric, xviii–xix; melancholic, xviii–xix; phlegmatic, xviii–xix; sanguine, xviii–xix
incubation period, 60
influenza: A, 12; A, epidemics of, 22–23; A, figure of, 14; B, 12, 66, 115; B, epidemics of, 23; C,12, 115; C, figure of, 16; classification of, 12–16; clinical diagnosis of, 71–79; complicated, 62–64; discovery of, 4–12, 115; dogs and, 29; eggs and, 73, 81, 82, 101, 115; envelope of, 13; extra-pulmonary complications of, 65–68, 108; felines and, 29; H1N1, 14, 24, 26, 53, 89, 93, 102, 108, 114, 115; H2N2, 24, 89, 114; H3N2, 14, 24, 89, 93, 102, 104, 114, 115; host responses to, 16–20; human shedding of, 17, 61, 68, 69, 70; important facts about, xxii; in children, 68–69; in chronic disease patients, 51, 69; in elderly patients, 69–70; in immunocompromised patients, 70; in pregnant women, 42–43, 70; manifestations in special populations, 68–70; morphology of, 12–16; naming of, 13; pathogenicity of, 16–20; pigs and, 8–9, 12, 116; poultry and, 27–30, 116, 117; prevention of, 41, 95–106, 109; prevention, figure of, 42; prevention, future research, 105–106; symptoms of, 60–70, 72–73, 76–77; symptoms, duration of, 60–61; transmission of, 3, 60; treatment of, 41, 85–95, 109; treatment, figure of, 86; treatment, future research, 105–106; treatment, supportive care, 87–88; uncomplicated, 60–62
Ivanovski, Dmitri, 114

Jenner, Edward, 98

Klimt, Gustav, 45
Koch, Robert, xvii, xx, 5, 7, 114; postulates of, xxi, 5, 7, 8, 114

laboratory testing, 79–84, 108; additional considerations, 84; culture 80–81; culture, conventional, 81; culture, figure of, 82; culture, rapid shell vial, 81; future development of, 84;

immunofluorescence microscopy, 83; nucleic acid testing, 83; rapid antigen tests, 81–83; serological tests, 83–84

Laidlaw, Patrick, 5, 11, 115

Leary, Timothy, 39

Lewis, David, 101–102

Lewis, Paul, 5, 8, 40

Livius, Titus, 111; *History of Rome*, 111

Lockwood, Harold, 41

malaria, 5, 7, 41

Mather, Cotton: quote from, 112

matrix proteins, 15, 88

McConnell, C.P., 85–86; *The Treatment of Influenza*, 85

Medical Research Council, 9, 10

Metropolitan Life Insurance Company, 32

miasma theory, xvii, xix–xx, 86

mumps, 10

Munch, Edvard, 46–47

myocarditis, 65

myositis, 66

Naeslund, Carl, 51

National Cancer Institute, 52

National Institute of Allergy and Infectious Diseases (NIAID), 55

National Institutes of Health (NIH), 51

National Institute for Medical Research, 9

Nicolle, Charles Jules Henry, 5, 7

Nightingale, Florence, xvii, xx

non-structural proteins, 15

nucleocapsid protein, 15

Olitsky, Peter K., 5, 6–7

Orthomyxoviridae, 13

oseltamivir. *See* antiviral medications

outbreak, 21; definition of, 22

pandemic, 23–25; definition of, 23; first documented, 112; measures of

preparation for, 25, 29, 54–57, 105–106, 109; of 1918, 31–54, 108; viruses causing, 26, 27–30, 109. *See also* avian influenza, H5N1

parasite, 2

Paris Peace Conference, 48

Pasteur, Louis, xvii, xx

Pasteur Institute, 5, 7

pasteurization, xx

patient interview. *See* health history

pericarditis, 65

Pfeiffer, Richard Friedrich Johannes, 4, 5, 7, 114; bacillus of, 4–5, 7, 8, 11, 50, 64, 114; bacillus, figure of, 6; phenomenon of, 7. *See also Bacillus influenzae* and *Haemophilius influenzae*

phages. *See* bacteriophages

Philadelphia, 37

Phillips: collection, 47–48; Duncan, 47–48; James, 47–48

physical examination, 71, 76–79, 108; patient etiquette for, 78

polio, 2, 3; vaccine for, 8

polymerase chain reaction (PCR), 53

polymerase proteins, 15

Porter, Katherine Anne, 38–39; *Pale Horse, Pale Rider*, 38–39

primary viral pneumonia, 62–64, 69, 70, 108; figure of, 63

Reeves, Richard: quote from, 21

Relenza®. *See* antiviral medications

respiratory syncytial virus, 23

Reye's syndrome, 66–67, 68, 84

ribonucleic acid (RNA), 3, 13, 108; catalytic, 3, 4; messenger, 3, 4; noncoding, 3, 4; proofreading of, 25, 108; ribosomal, 3, 4; transfer, 3, 4

ribosomes, 4

rimantadine, 29

ringworm, 2

Rockefeller Institute for Medical Research, 5, 6, 8, 10, 40

Roosevelt, Franklin D., 35
Russian flu, 114, 115

San Francisco, 40
San Quentin Prison, 32
Santayana, George, 54
scabies, 2
Schiele, Egon, 45–46; self-portrait of, 46
secondary bacterial pneumonia, 50, 64, 69, 70, 108
Seymour, Charles, 48
Shope, Richard, 5, 8–9, 11–12, 40, 50, 64, 102, 107, 114; figure of, 9
Shotwell, James T., 48
sialic acid, 14; receptors of, 28
Simon, Sir John, xvii, xx
smallpox, 95–98; flat, 96; hemorrhagic, 96; modified, 96; modified, figure of, 97; ordinary, 96; vaccination, 96–97. *See also Variola*
Smith, Wilson, 5, 11, 115
Southgate, M. Therese, 46–47; *The Cover*, 46–47
Spanish flu, 21, 24, 32, 114
Starr, Isaac, 43–44; *Influenza in 1918*, 43–44
Sweeney, Frederick, 59–60
Swift, Homer, 10
swine flu, 8, 11, 26, 101–104, 114, 115, 116; immunization program, 102–104, 115; immunization program, figure of, 103
Symmetrel®. *See* antiviral medications

T-lymphocytes: CD4, 19; CD8, 19
Tamiflu®. *See* antiviral medications
Taubenberger, Jeffrey, 31, 52–53; quote from, 31
Taylor, R. M., 115
thymine, 3
toxic shock syndrome (TSS), 67–68
transverse myelitis, 66
Treaty of Versailles, 48
tuberculosis, xx, 8

United Kingdom Health Protection, 117
United States Department of Health and Human Services (HHS), 55
uracil, 3

vaccination, xxi, 39–40, 95–104, 107; benefits of, 98–99; figure of, 99, 103; future research, 105–106; killed virus (TIV), 100–101; killed virus, side effects of, 100–101; live virus (LAIV), 101; live virus, side effects of, 101; recommendations for, 69, 70; swine flu, 101–104
vaccinia, 10
Variola, 95–96; figure of, 96; major, 95–96; minor, 95–96. *See also* smallpox
variolation, 97–98
Vaughan, Roscoe, 53
virus: classification of, 3; definition of, 1–4; envelope of, 2, 3; morphology of, 3; origin of, 2; origin of name, xxi; replication, 3–4, 107; transcription, 3; translation, 3, 4
Voltaire. *See* Arouet, François-Marie
von Liebig, Justus, xvii, xx

Wilson, Woodrow, 32, 48
Wolfe, Benjamin, 62–64
Wolfe, Thomas, 62–64; *Look Homeward, Angel*, 63–64
World Health Organization (WHO), xxii, 25, 27, 56–57, 98, 109, 117
World Organization for Animal Health (OIE), 56
World War I, 32–35, 48, 49; figure of, 35, 36

yellow fever, 8

zanamivir. *See* antiviral medications

About the Author

RONI K. DEVLIN M.D. is an Infectious Diseases physician at Mercy Health Partners in Muskegon, Michigan. She received her medical degree from the University of Colorado, and returned to her home state of Michigan to complete a combined residency in both Internal Medicine and Pediatrics. She then finished her subspecialty training in Infectious Diseases at Dartmouth. She now resides in Grand Rapids, Michigan, where she divides her time between the practice of medicine and the world of bookselling as the owner of Literary Life Bookstore & More, Inc.